Dental Techniques

A Colour Atlas of

Acid Etch Technique

Professor John J. Murray

PhD, MChD, FDSRCS (Eng)

Head of the Department of Child Dental Health, Dental School, University of Newcastle upon Tyne, and Honorary Consultant, Newcastle Health Authority

T. Gordon Bennett

BDS, FDS, DOrth RCS (Eng)

Consultant Orthodontist, Newcastle Health Authority, and Honorary Clinical Lecturer, University of Newcastle upon Tyne

Wolfe Medical Publications Ltd

Published by Wolfe Medical Publications Ltd, 1984
Printed by Royal Smeets Offset b.v.,
Weert, Netherlands
ISBN 07234 1014 3

This book is one of the titles in the series of Wolfe Dental Techniques, a series which will eventually cover a wide range of subjects.

If you wish to be kept informed of new additions to the series and receive details of our other titles, please write to
Wolfe Medical Publications Ltd, Wolfe House,
3 Conway Street, London W1P 6HE

A few of the other titles in print and in preparation in the Dental Techniques series

Technique of Complete Denture Construction
Partial Denture Design
Wisdom Tooth Surgery
Apicectomy
Surgery of the Temporomandibular Joint
Dental Occlusion
Periodontology
Pre-prosthetic Oral Surgery
Endodontic Surgery

Dedication
To Valerie, Mark, Christopher, and Sheila, Catherine, Jenny.

Acknowledgements

Almost all of the photographs in this Atlas were taken at the Dental School and Hospital, Newcastle upon Tyne; we would like to pay tribute to Mr B. Hill, Senior Photographer, and his staff for their skilful assistance and willing co-operation. We are grateful to Dr P.H. Gordon for his constructive comments on the manuscript, to Mr A.W.G. Walls for his help in providing some of the photographs, particularly the Duralingual acid etch retained bridge and the electron photomicrographs, and to Mr D. Penketh for Figures **242** and **243.** The first four figures are reproduced by kind permission of Dr B.F. Williams, Institute of Dental Surgery, London. We would like to thank Mrs G. Rowley and Mrs V. Dyer for their secretarial assistance.

Contents

(i)

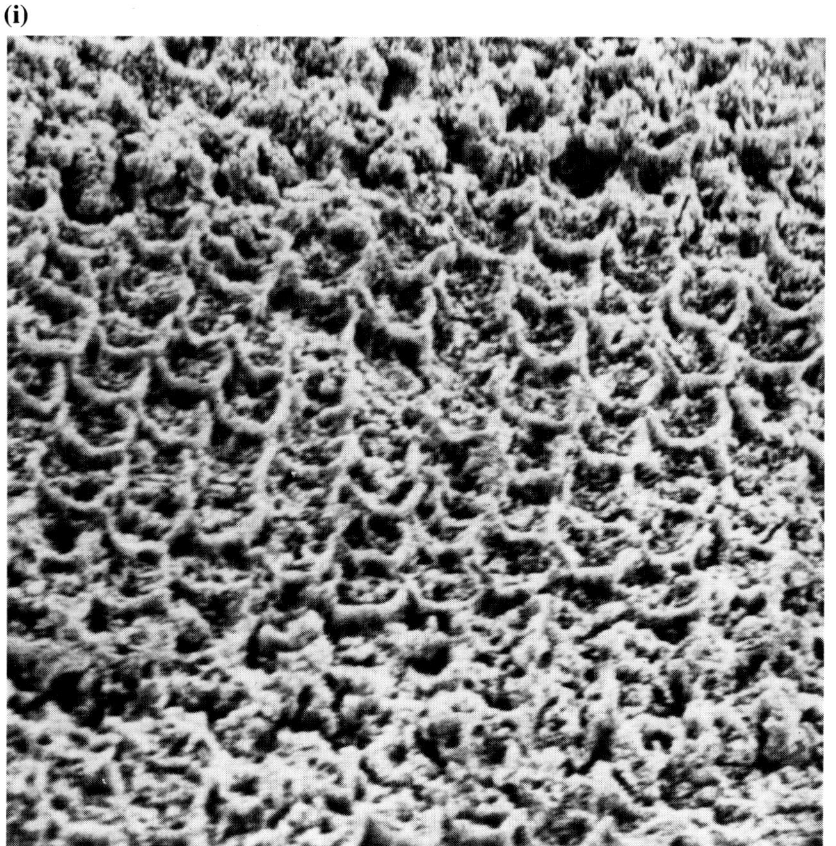

(i) Acid etched enamel. An electron photomicrograph (× 1000) of the surface of enamel, etched for 60 seconds with 37 per cent orthophosphoric acid, showing the prism boundaries in relief.

(ii)

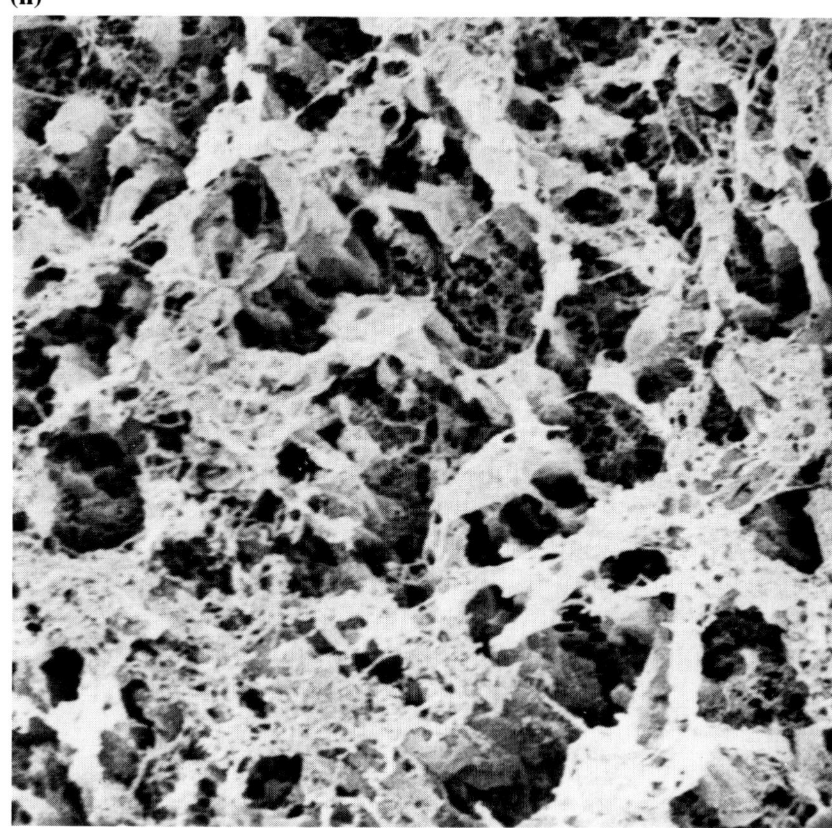

(ii) The 'fitting surface' of a fissure sealant. An electron photomicrograph (× 1000) of the resin tags of a fissure sealant applied to a premolar tooth. The enamel was removed by applying Calex, a mixture of concentrated hydrochloric acid and ethylene diamine tetra acetic acid (EDTA) for 24 hours.

Development of fissure sealants

The desire to find a material that would adhere directly onto enamel has been like the alchemist's search for a method of turning base metal into gold. During the 20th century silver nitrate, black copper cement, zinc ferrocyanide and methyl-2-cyano-acrylate were all tried, unsuccessfully, in an attempt to find a material that would stick permanently to the occlusal surfaces of posterior teeth and prevent occlusal caries. Ideally, what is required is a material which is runny enough so that, when applied, it runs into all the nooks and crannies and blocks the fissures of the occlusal surface; it then must set quickly, adhere to the enamel surface and be strong enough to withstand masticatory forces. These major requirements were fulfilled with the introduction of the acid etch technique, in which the enamel surface is roughened with acid, and the development of various materials based on the Bis GMA resin originally reported by Bowen. A number of methods have been developed to polymerise or cure the resin; first ultraviolet light, then chemical activation. More recently visible light has been used enabling fissure sealing to be carried out more quickly and easily. However, the basic procedure for successful fissure sealing has remained essentially unchanged since 1970:

1 Clean the occlusal surface with pumice or an oil free, fluoride free paste.
2 Wash and dry the tooth.
3 Apply acid etchant (30 to 60 per cent phosphoric acid) to the occlusal surface with a cottonwool pledget or brush for 60 seconds.
4 Wash thoroughly with water.
5 Dry for 30 seconds.
6 Apply sealant.
7 Polymerise material.
8 Check occlusion.

The first ultraviolet light used to polymerise a fissure sealant was extremely bulky. This was soon replaced by a much neater piece of equipment which was easier to use and could rest on the cusp of a tooth, while the agent was polymerised for 60 seconds. This method gained popularity in the early 1970s and came to be known as the 'ray gun', but the initial cost of the UV light was a drawback.

Caution

All etching solutions contain acid, usually phosphoric acid. Avoid contact with eyes, skin, oral mucosa and dentine. In case of contact, wash immediately with water and seek medical attention if eyes are involved. Do not take internally.

Composite materials contain polymerisable monomers which may cause sensitisation or irritation if allowed to contact soft tissues. Wash thoroughly with soap and water if contact occurs. Do not use if there is a known allergy to methacrylate resin.

1 An example of the first ultraviolet light used to cure fissure sealants.

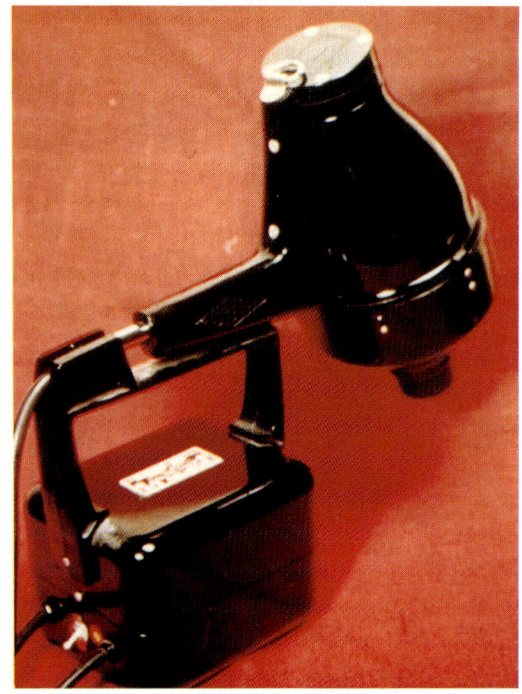

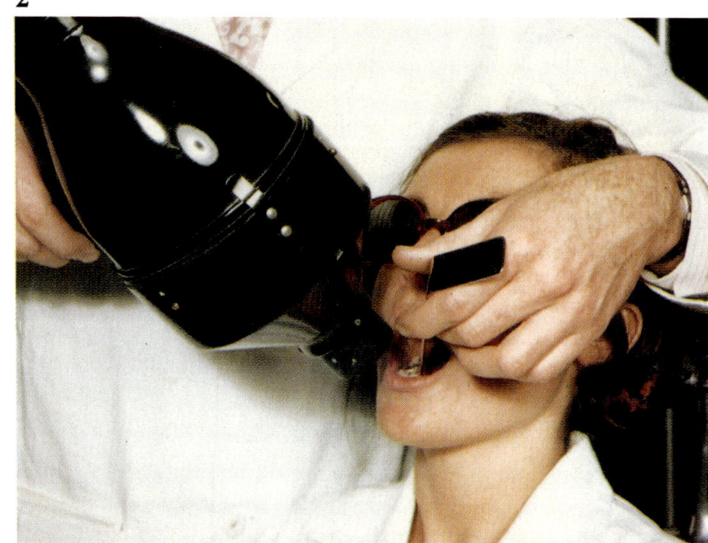

2 The difficulty of using this light source in the mouth.

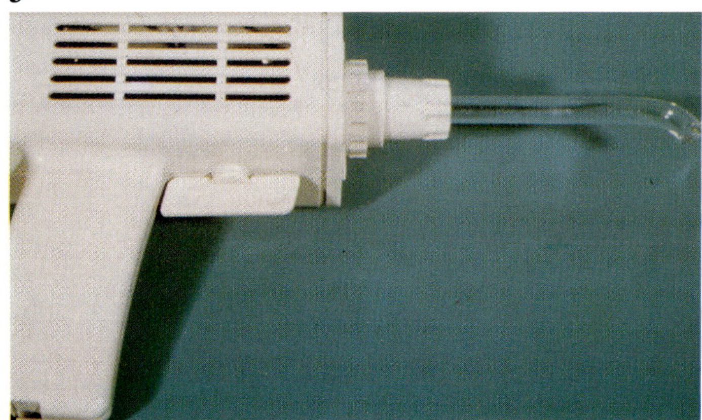

3 The specially developed Nuva-lite.

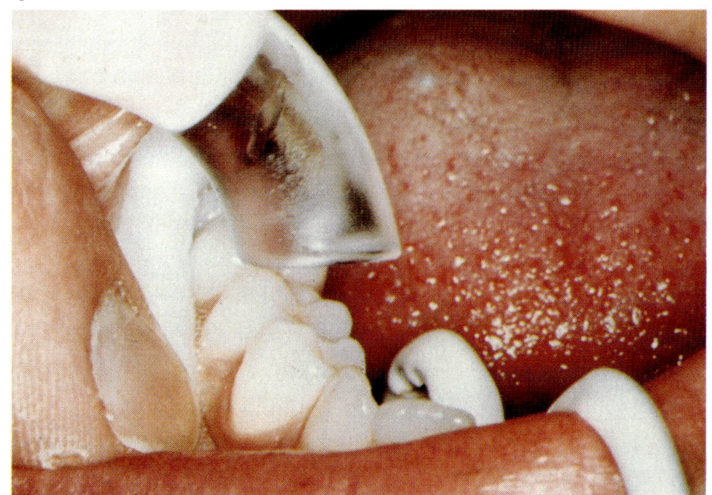

4 The tip of the light resting on the cusp of a tooth.

A number of methods involving chemical polymerisation were developed, for example Concise White Sealant^{R} and Delton^{R}. Polymerisation was achieved by mixing one drop of 'universal' liquid and one drop of catalyst together and waiting for chemical polymerisation to occur. The application technique was broadly similar for both materials.

5

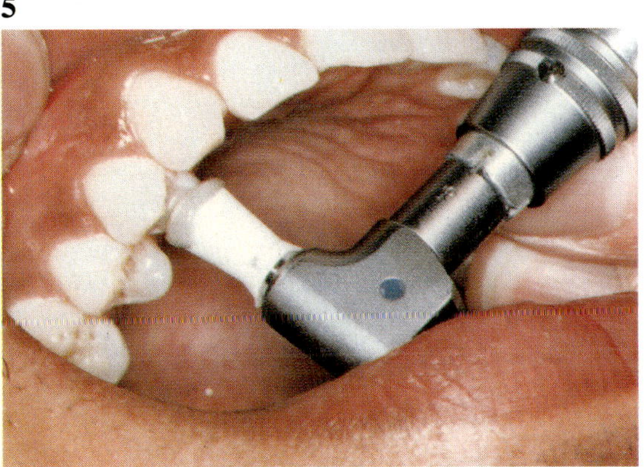

5 Clean the occlusal surface with pumice or other oil free, fluoride free prophylaxis paste.

6

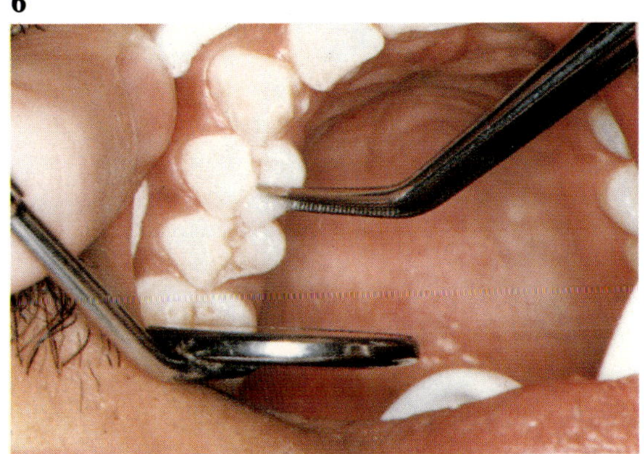

6 Apply acid etching liquid (tooth conditioner) to the occlusal surface with a cottonwool pledget or brush for 60 seconds.

7

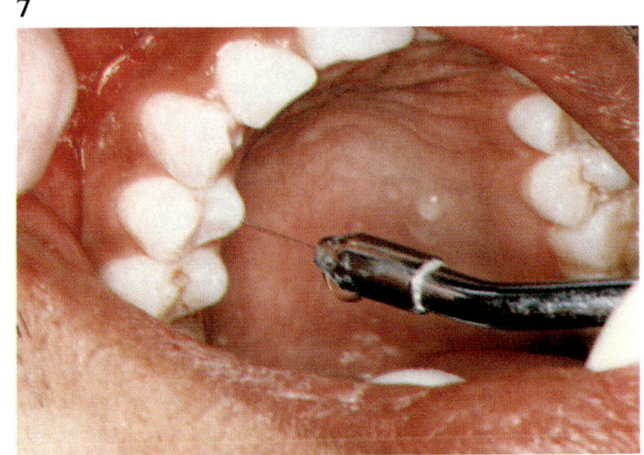

7 Then wash thoroughly with water.

8

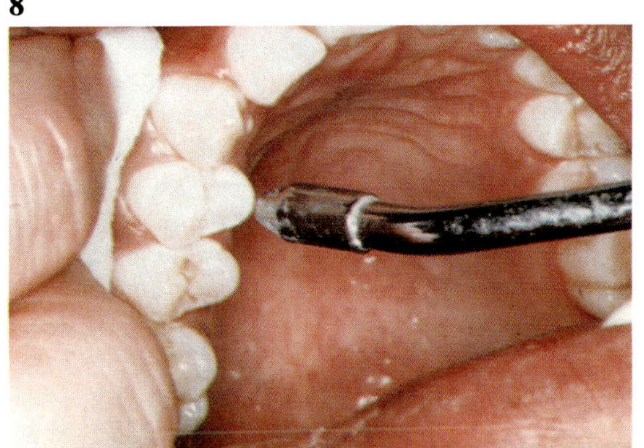

8 Dry with compressed air for 30 seconds. Inspect the surface. If it does not appear 'frosty' re-etch. The tooth must be dry.

9

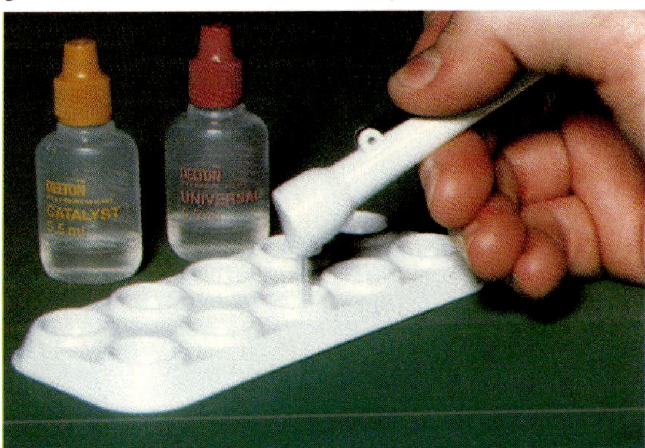

9 Mix sealant – one drop of 'universal' and one drop of catalyst – in a mixing well.

10

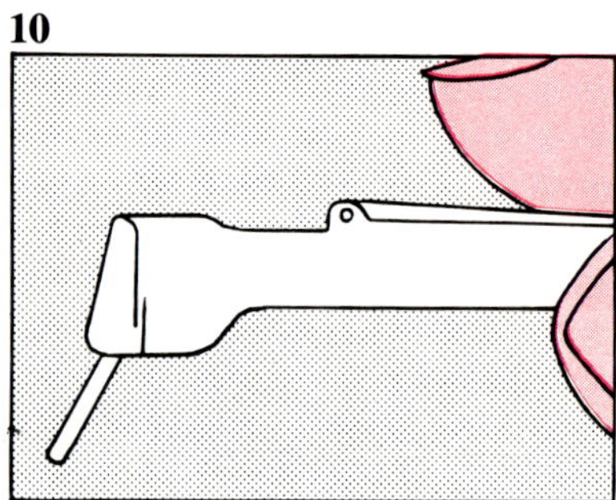

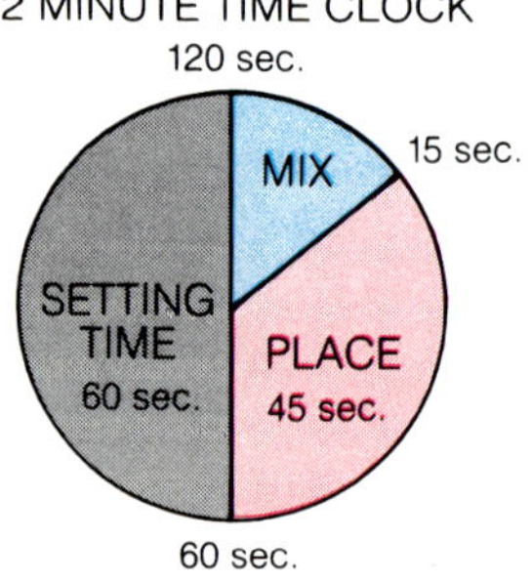

10 Apply sealant with applicator and wait for chemical polymerisation to take place – the time cycle is approximately two minutes.

(This applicator is a patent protected design of Johnson & Johnson.)

11

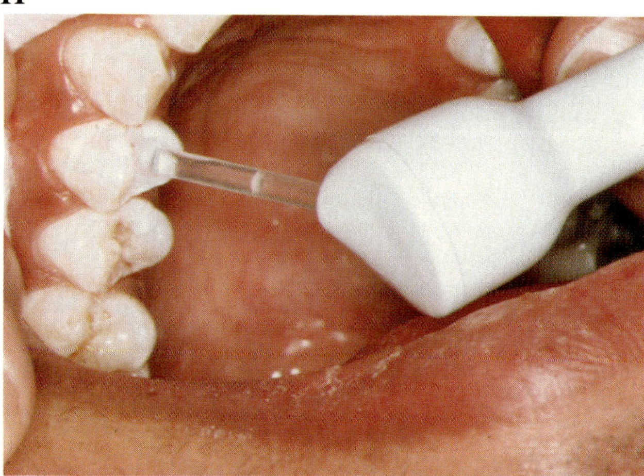

11 Sealant being applied.

13

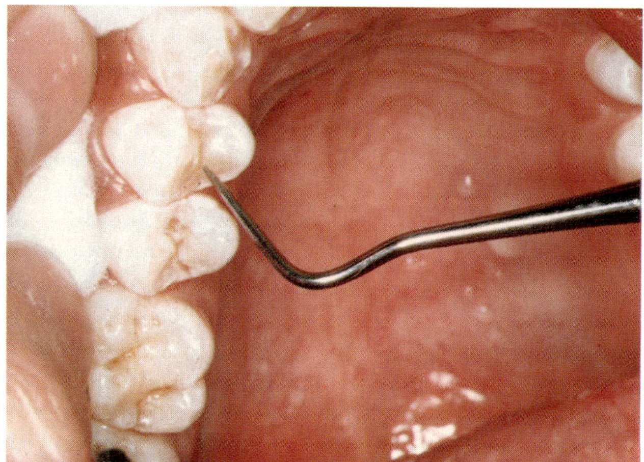

13 Check occlusal surface for coverage and retention.

12

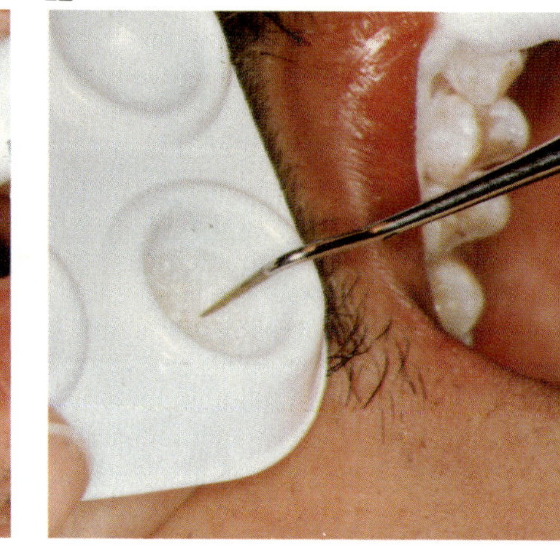

12 Check to ensure the sealant has polymerised in the mixing well.

The chemical method of polymerisation eliminated the need for an ultraviolet light source, but the polymerisation period took at least one minute, during which time the tooth had to remain dry. Sometimes this was not possible to achieve, particularly for newly erupted first permanent molar teeth, right at the back of the mouth, in young children.

The third method of polymerisation, by blue visible light, has reduced the curing time to 20 seconds. A device is incorporated into the Prisma[R] light system which emits a short buzzing sound every 10 seconds. The cleaning, washing, and etching procedures are identical to those previously described.

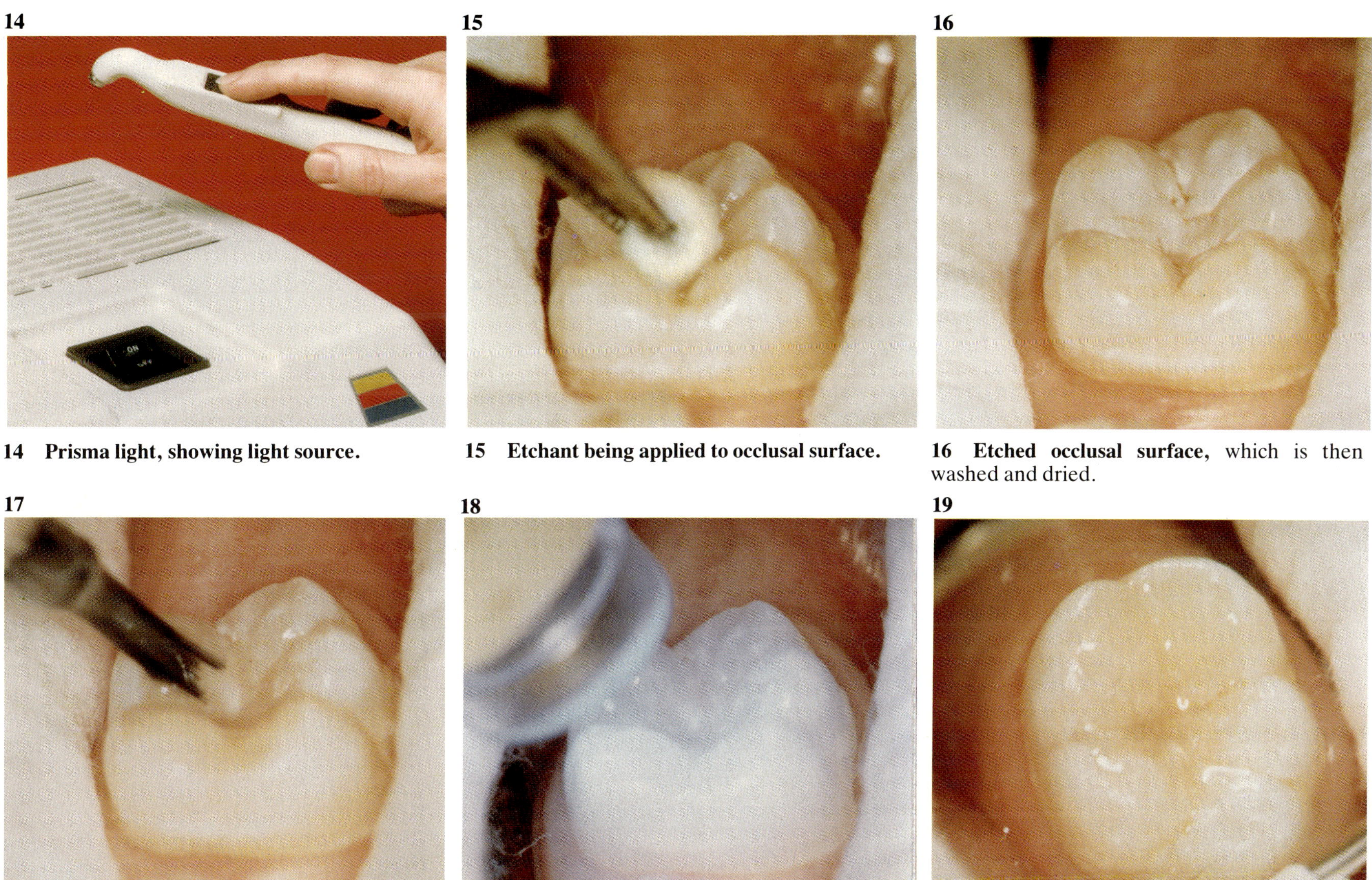

14 Prisma light, showing light source.

15 Etchant being applied to occlusal surface.

16 Etched occlusal surface, which is then washed and dried.

17 Following washing and drying, Prisma-shield[R] is applied to the occlusal surface with a brush.

18 Material is cured for 20 seconds.

19 Mirror view showing fissure sealant in place.

There is no doubt that the advent of fissure sealants has changed attitudes to the 'early carious lesion'. At one time it used to be regarded as inevitable that caries would occur sooner or later on the occlusal surface of molar and premolar teeth. The concept of 'prophylactic odontotomy' promulgated by Thaddeus P. Hyatt in the 1920s was that it was better to restore the tooth with amalgam before caries actually occurred, thus preventing larger lesions from developing later. However, many young children find the process of drilling and filling unpleasant and the 'ideal' restoration which never fails from marginal leakage is difficult if not impossible to achieve. The concept of 'prophylactic odontotomy' or 'preventive filling' was certainly responsible for unnecessary restorative procedures being applied to millions of teeth. When fissure sealants are applied correctly to the surfaces of teeth with a high potential for decay, particularly the occlusal surface of permanent molars, the chances of maintaining the dentition completely free from caries or fillings are greatly increased.

20

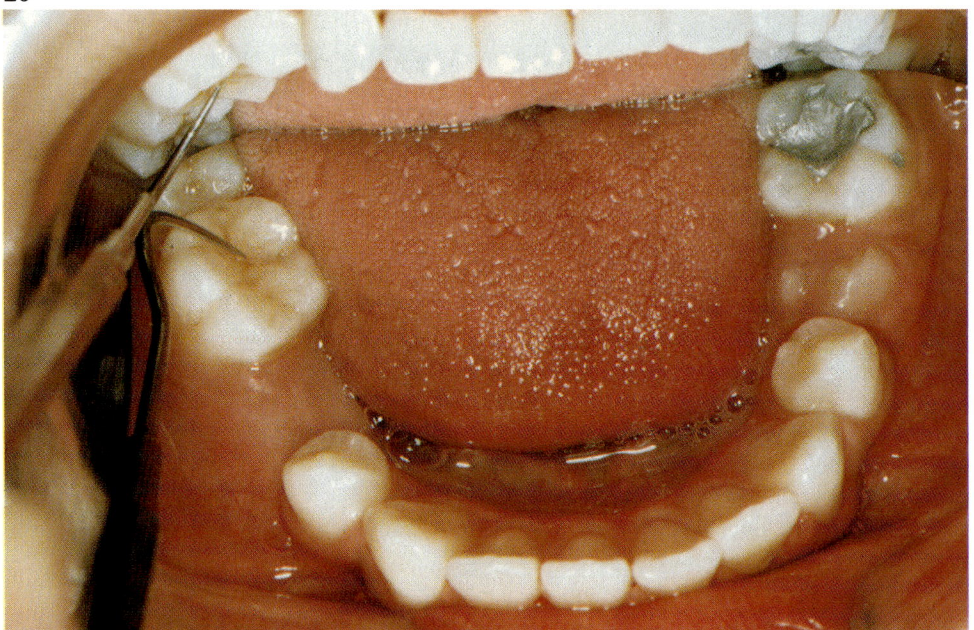

20 A child who has an extensive restoration on the occlusal surface of the lower left first permanent molar. The margin of the restoration is defective around the distobuccal cusp. The cavity will have to be enlarged and the restoration renewed.

The lower right first permanent molar has been fissure sealed successfully. This not only means that a restoration has been prevented, but also that the 'repair of repair' has also been prevented.

New approach to restoring children's teeth

When caries has penetrated the enamel and reached the amelodentinal junction, irreversible destruction has occurred and the potential for the carious lesion to spread along the amelodentinal junction and into dentine increases. The only treatment is to drill out the decay and place a restoration. Traditionally, the outline of the cavity preparation following Black's directives on classical cavity preparation in the 1880s has involved the concept of 'extension for prevention' in that the occlusal fissures are included in the cavity preparation, and the cavity is undercut, in the hope that the ensuing amalgam restoration will prevent the recurrence of caries. This method results inevitably in a certain amount of sound tooth tissue being removed. However, it is now possible in early carious lesions which have just penetrated into dentine to remove the caries with minimal cavity preparation, to protect the exposed dentine with a calcium hydroxide preparation and then to acid etch the cavity and the occlusal surface in exactly the same way as for fissure sealing. Then the cavity is filled with a composite material, which has the same chemical composition as a fissure sealant, but with silica particles added to give greater strength. The occlusal surface is then fissure sealed with an unfilled resin and the whole surface, including the small pit defect, is polymerised. The ensuing restoration is simpler for the patient and embodies the principle of extension for prevention without the unnecessary removal of sound tissue.

21

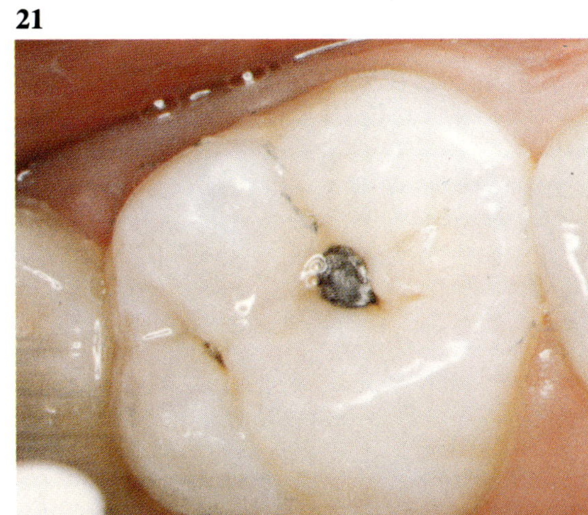

21 An upper left first permanent molar with a small amalgam restoration in the mesial pit and an early carious lesion in the distal pit.

22

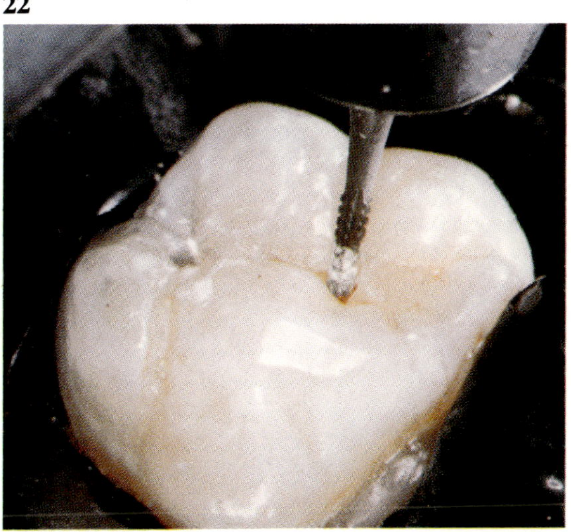

22 A fine bur is used to remove the carious tissue and deficient amalgam from the tooth, which is isolated by means of a rubber dam or cotton rolls.

23

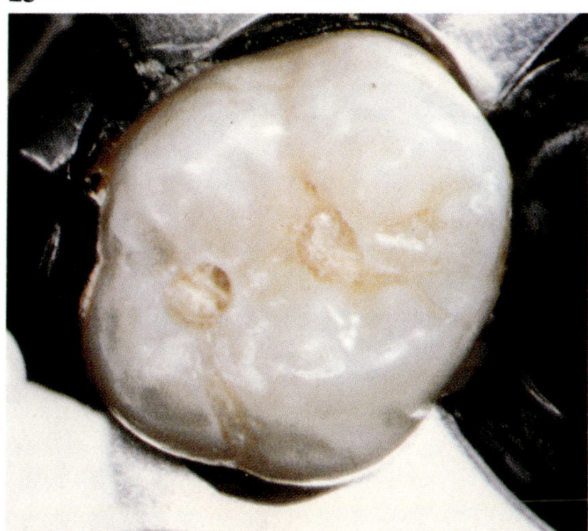

23 A view of the cavities. The floor of each cavity is then lined with a calcium hydroxide preparation.

24

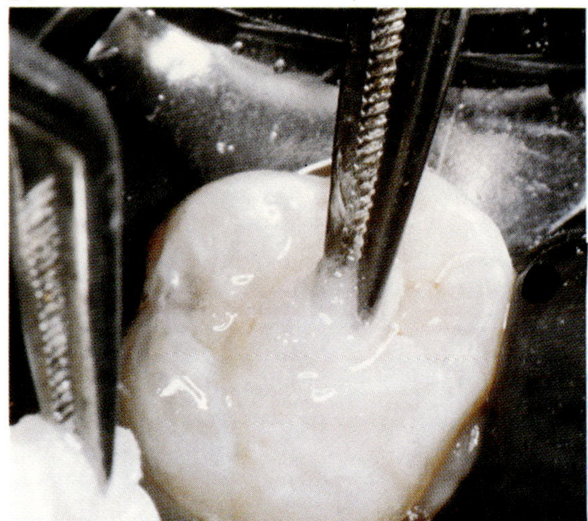

24 The walls of the cavities, and the whole of the occlusal surface are etched for 60 seconds.

25

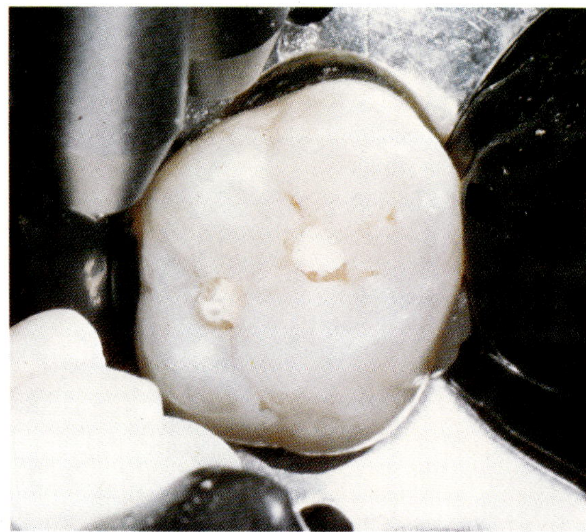

25 The cavities and occlusal surface are then washed for 10 seconds and dried for 30 seconds to obtain a 'frosty' appearance.

26

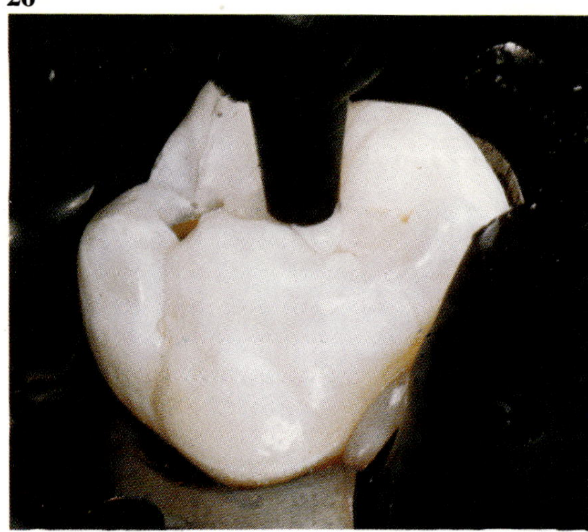

26 The cavities are filled with a light sensitive 'filled composite resin' (and . . .

27

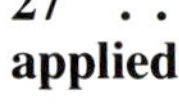

27 . . . a light sensitive fissure sealant is then applied to the occlusal surface.

28

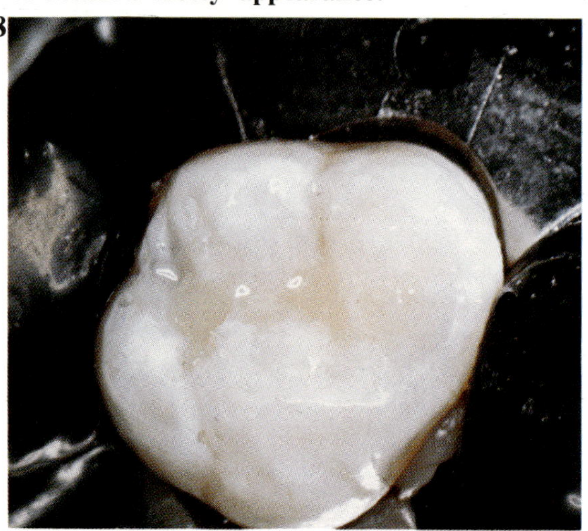

28 The material is then cured for 20–30 seconds with a suitable light to complete the restoration.

29

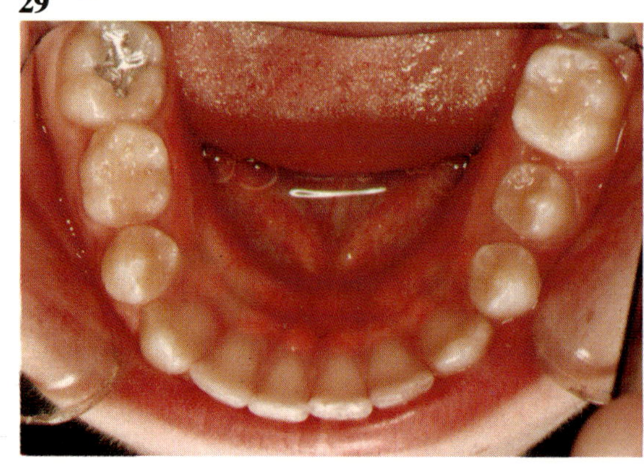

29 A view of the lower arch of another patient showing a composite restoration and fissure sealant on the lower left first permanent molar compared with a conventional amalgam restoration on the lower right first permanent molar.

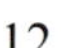

Restoration of fractured incisors

When a tooth is fractured, particularly if dentine is exposed, the vitality of the pulp of the tooth is at much greater risk, because it has lost part of the very hard protective outer covering. Even if the tooth is kept clean, the loss of hard tissue following a crown fracture means that the pulp is now subjected to greater thermal and chemical changes than would otherwise be the case. This increases the risk of pulp death in a fractured tooth. The treatment of choice is to cover the exposed dentine as quickly as possible so as to try and maintain the vitality of the tooth. Before the introduction of the acid etch technique, the only method available was by cementing a stainless steel band or crown on the tooth in the hope that the pulp could be protected until root formation had been completed. Then the tooth could eventually be restored with a crown, usually of porcelain, when the patient was about 16 years of age.

The advent of the acid etch technique meant that a tooth coloured material could be bonded on to the fractured area, thereby replacing the lost tooth tissue. At first, this method was regarded as a most helpful, but temporary, method and it was assumed that the final restoration would still be a porcelain jacket crown. During the last 10 to 15 years a number of modifications have been suggested to the technique and there have been considerable improvements in the aesthetics of composite materials, so the acid etch technique for restoring fractured incisors should now be regarded as a medium to long-term treatment and in some cases the definitive restoration.

30

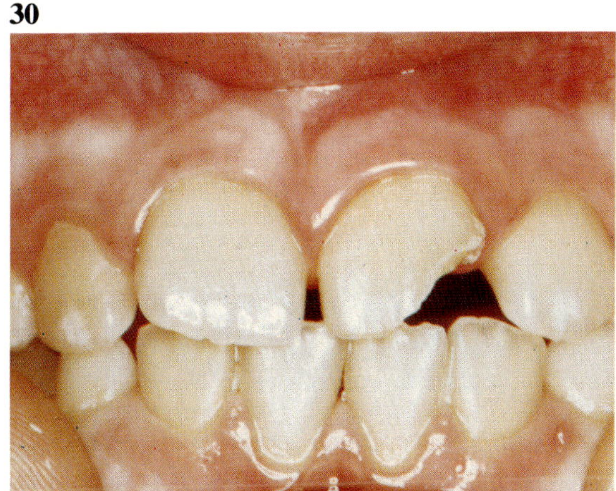

30 The upper left central incisor has been fractured, exposing dentine.

31

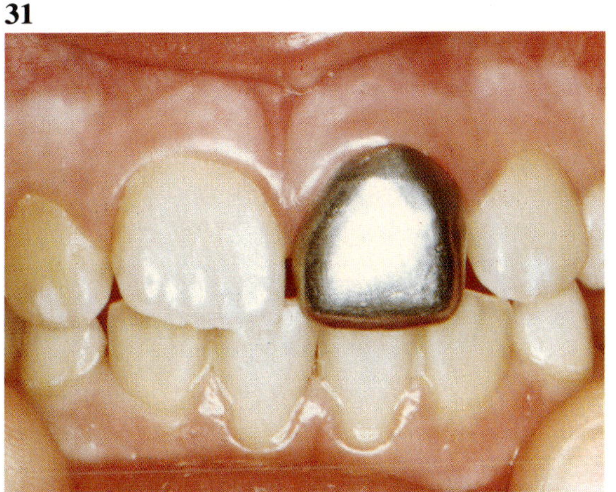

31 The traumatised tooth is covered with a stainless steel crown.

32

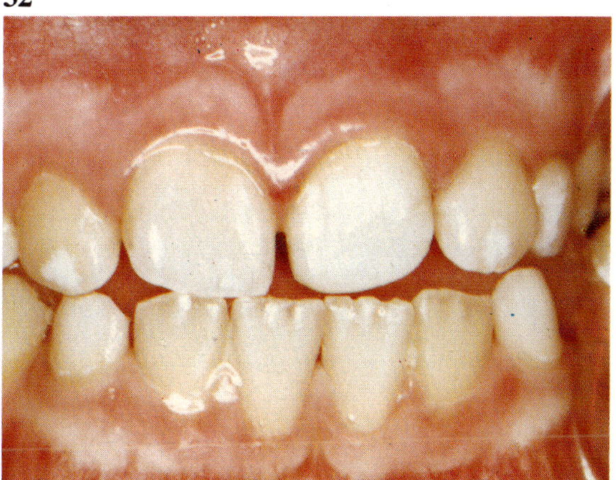

32 The tooth restored (in 1972) with an acid etch composite restoration.

The following technique has been employed for the restoration of fractured permanent incisors in young children aged 6 to 10 years, who present having recently been in an accident. The method is suitable for fractures in which dentine is involved, but the pulp should not be exposed. In these cases the prime objective is to try to preserve the vitality of the pulp so that root development will continue normally.

33

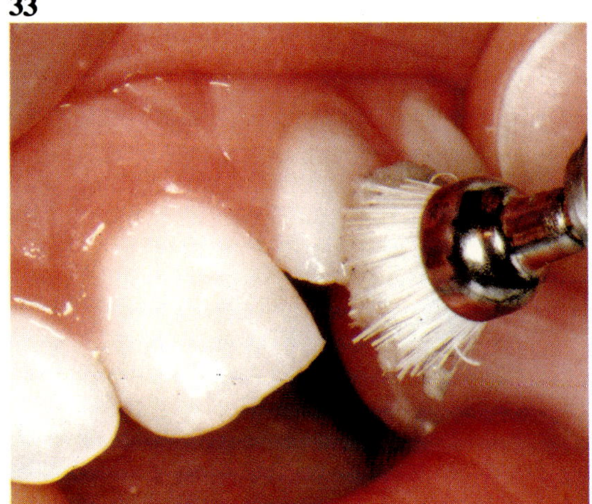

33 The tooth is cleaned with pumice.

34

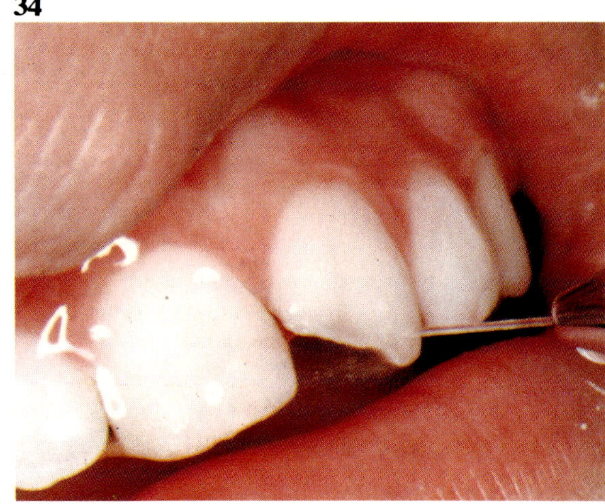

34 The tooth is washed and dried.

35

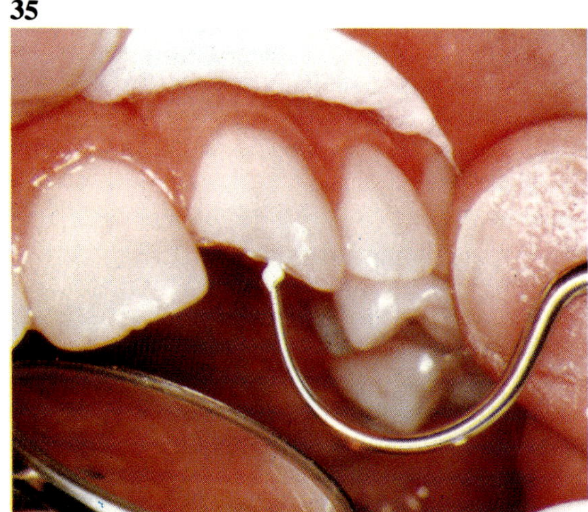

35 The exposed dentine is protected with a calcium hydroxide preparation.

36

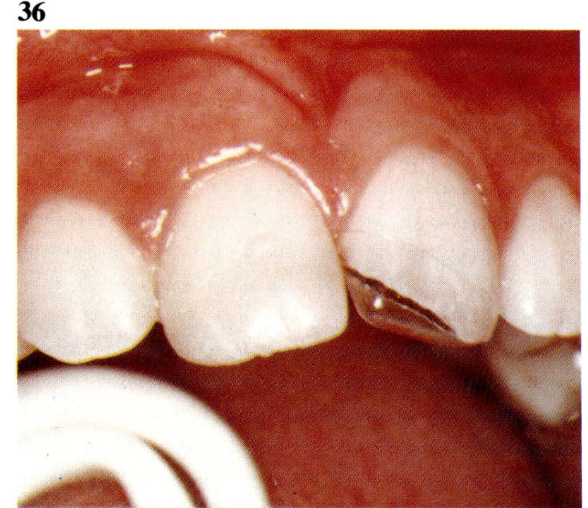

36 A crown former is trimmed so that it forms a matrix which just covers the fracture line and extends 2 to 3mm onto the remaining crown labially and palatally. It is essential that the crown former fits tightly onto the tooth.

37

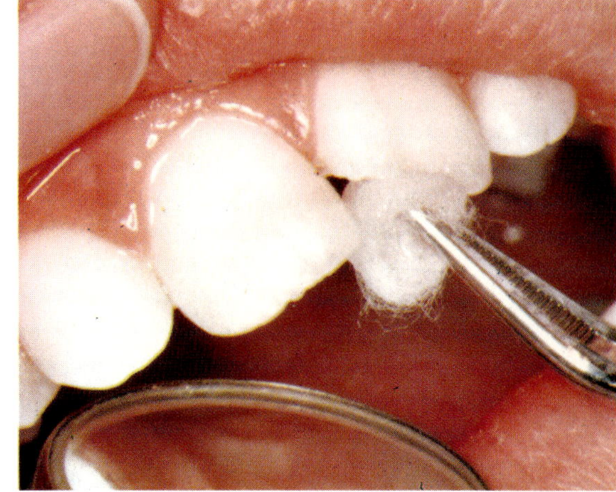

37 The fractured enamel, and 2 to 3mm only of normal enamel, labially and palatally, is etched for 60 seconds. Note that no preparation of the fractured enamel has been carried out.

38

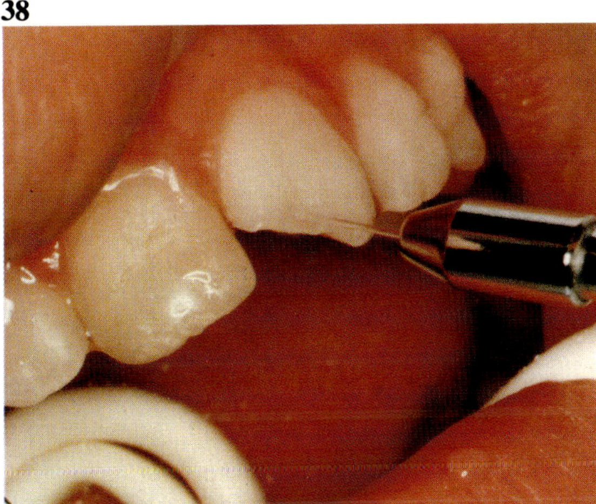

38 The tooth is washed for 10 seconds.

39

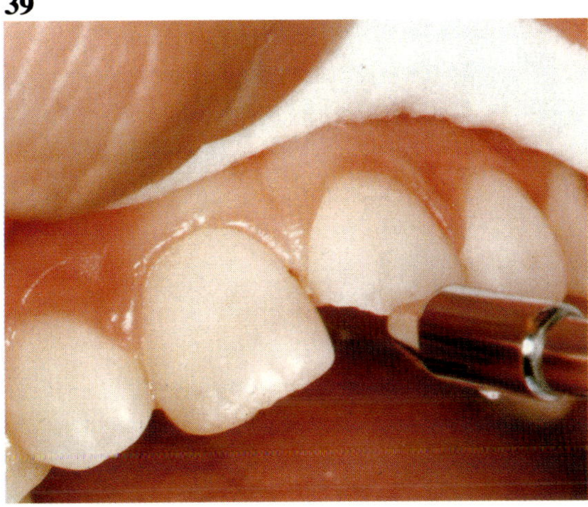

39 The tooth is dried for 30 seconds until the 'frosty' appearance is seen.

40

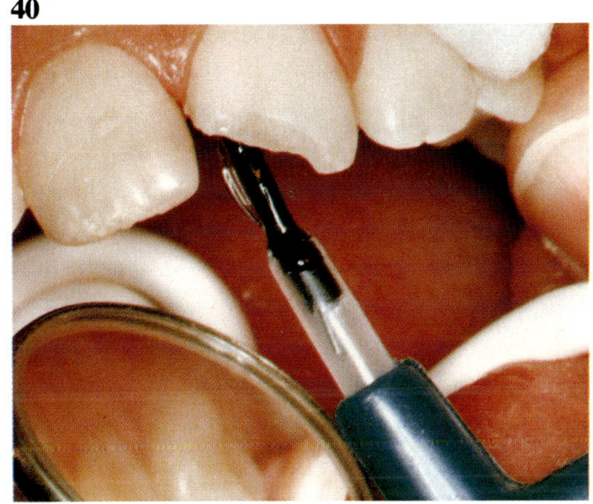

40 The fracture line is painted with bonding agent.

41

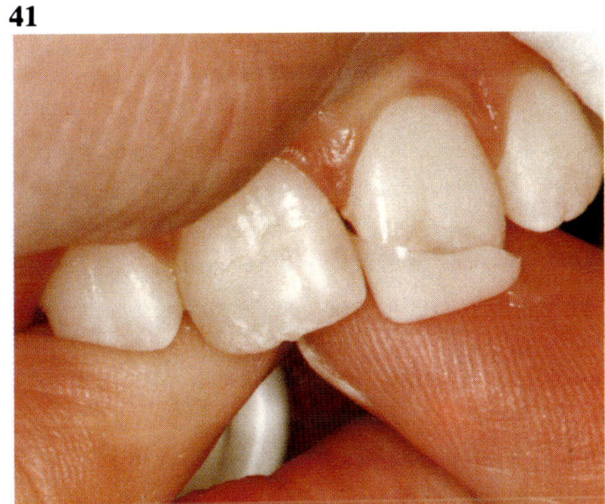

41 The composite is mixed, placed in the crown former, and held firmly on the tooth for 5 minutes.

42

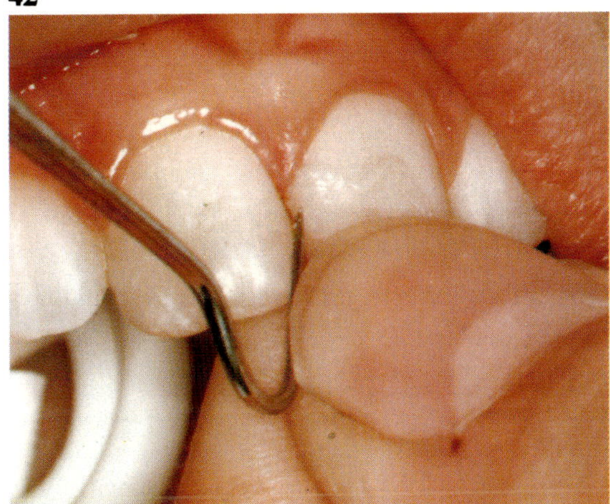

42 Allowing the composite to set. Although some excess can be removed from the labial surface with a probe, it is essential that the finger and thumb holding the crown former onto the tooth do not move and that pressure is maintained on the crown for 5 minutes to allow chemical polymerisation to take place. If the composite is disturbed during the setting reaction the strength of the bond will be diminished and a smooth polished finish to the surface of the composite will not be obtained.

43

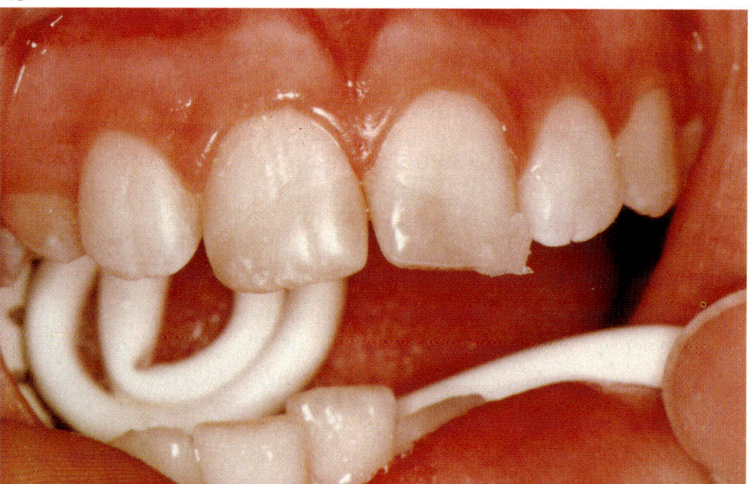

43 After 5 minutes the finger pressure is removed.

44

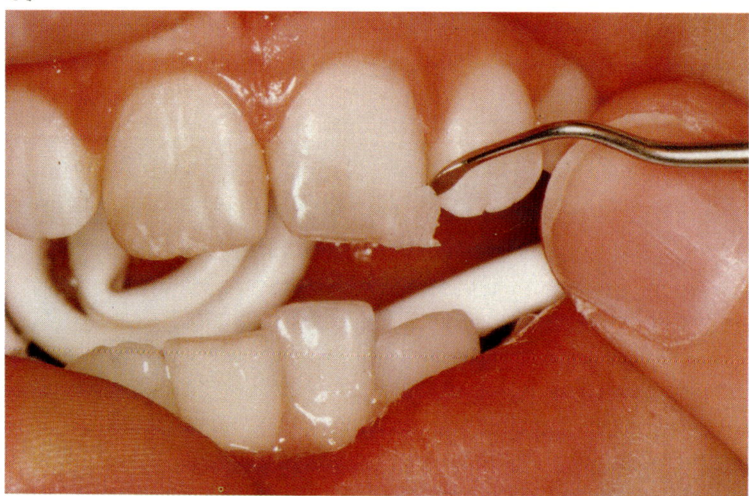

44 Excess composite is removed with an excavator. This is simple to do providing the acid etching has extended only to the margin of the crown former.

45

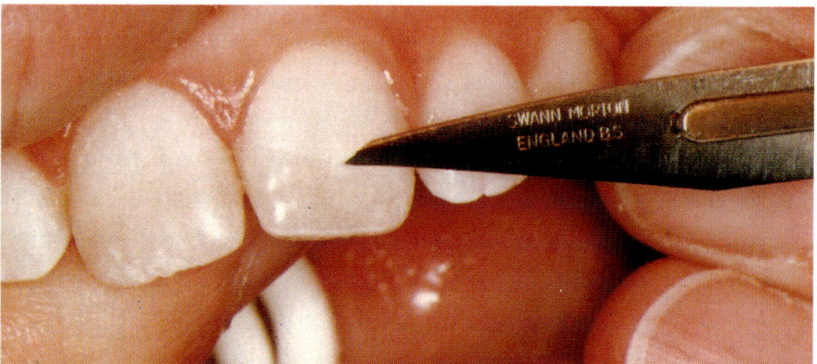

45 The celluloid crown is removed with a scalpel. Any excess composite is removed with a rotary instrument. If at all possible the labial surface is not touched, as the fine smooth surface obtained by contact with the celluloid crown former is extremely difficult to reproduce, even if a glaze is applied.

46

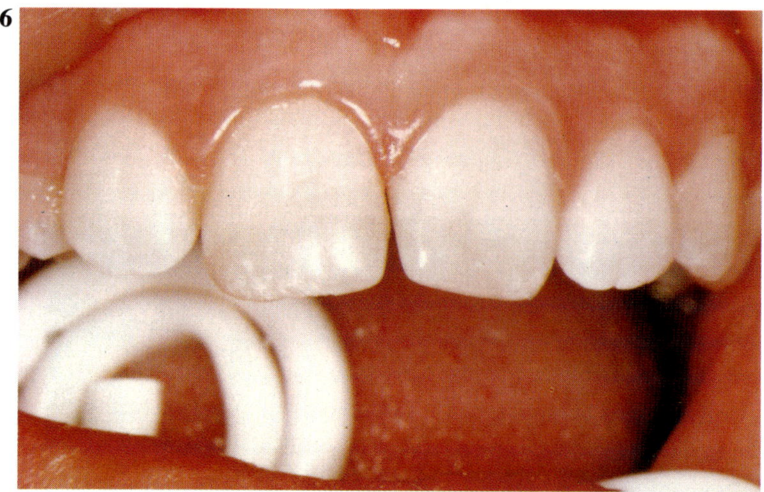

46 The final restoration should approximate to the original crown shape. It will be noted that there is a similar restoration on the other central incisor.

The final restoration should approximate to the original shape. The treatment is simple and the principles are essentially the same as for the fissure sealant technique. The main purpose, that of protecting the pulp, has been achieved with no tooth preparation, with considerably better aesthetics than the stainless steel crown. One disadvantage of the method described is that marginal staining can occur, particularly on the labial surface where the composite restoration overlapped 2 to 3mm onto normal enamel. If the stain occurs it can be polished away at a recall visit. Some operators recommend bevelling the fractured enamel or cutting a 'half enamel preparation' in an attempt to achieve greater thickness of composite and reduce the marginal staining. An example of the bevelled enamel technique, using light sensitive composite resin, will now be shown.

47

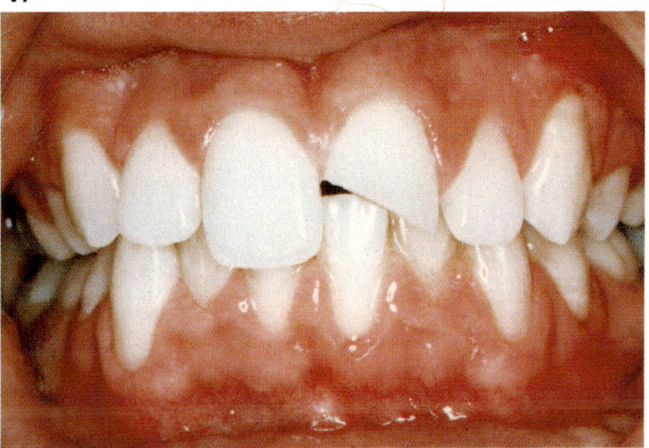

47 A fracture of the upper left central incisor, in a 15-year-old patient, involving enamel and dentine.

48

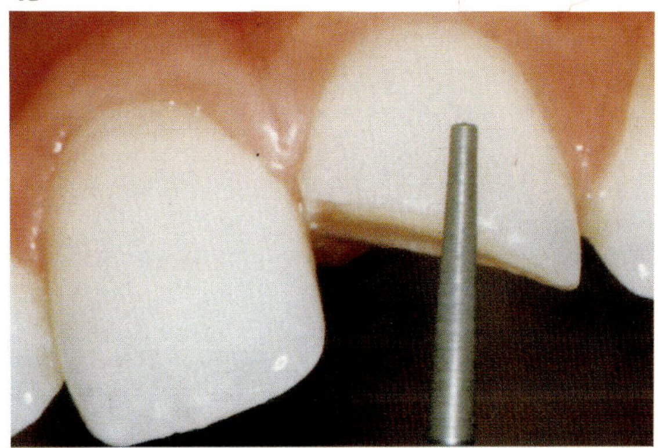

48 A tapered diamond bur is used to produce a bevel at an angle of approximately 45° to the labial surface.

49

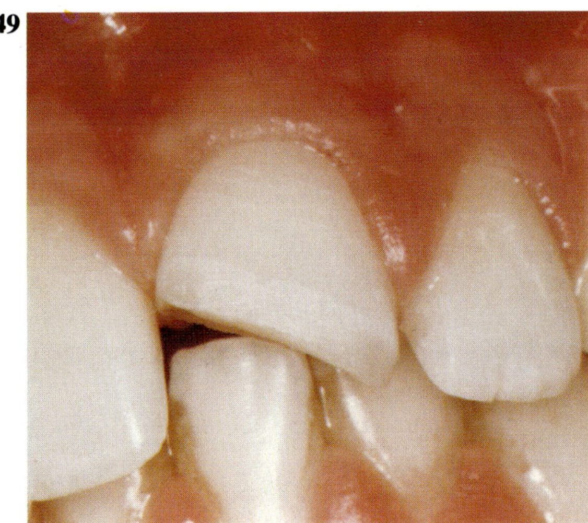

49 The bevel extends 2 to 3mm up the labial surface, beyond the line of the fracture.

50

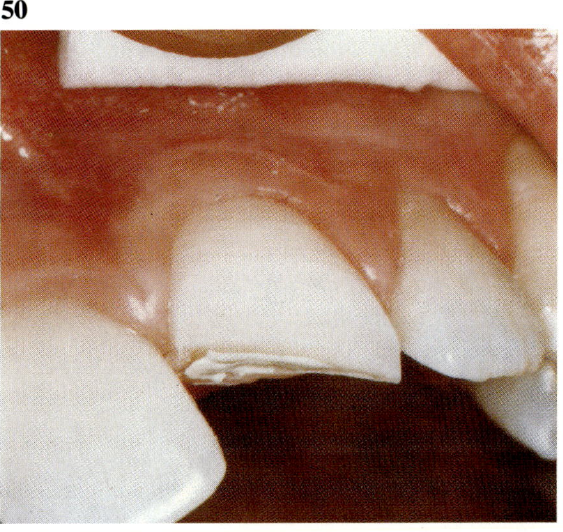

50 The dentine is protected with a calcium hydroxide preparation and the tooth is etched, washed and dried so as to obtain a 'frosty' appearance.

51

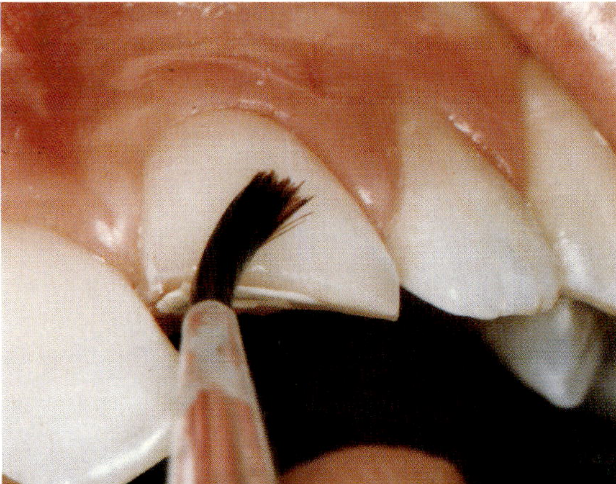

51 Bonding agent is applied with a brush.

52

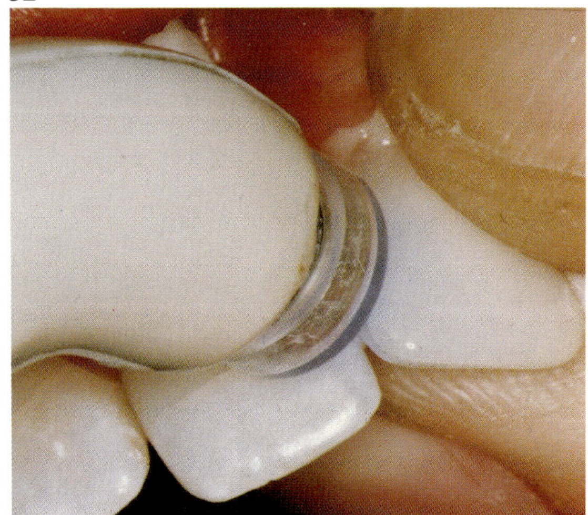

52 The crown former is filled with light sensitive composite resin and placed in position. Excess material is removed with a plastic instrument and the material is cured with the light source. Both labial and palatal surfaces should be cured to ensure polymerisation.

53

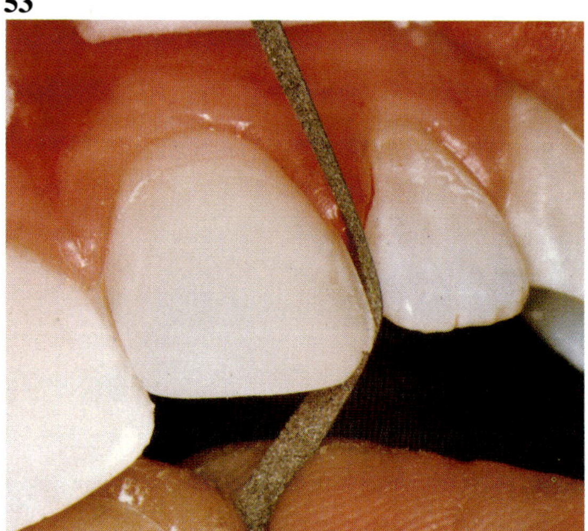

53 The crown former is removed and the margins smoothed by means of a Swift[R] abrasive strip

54

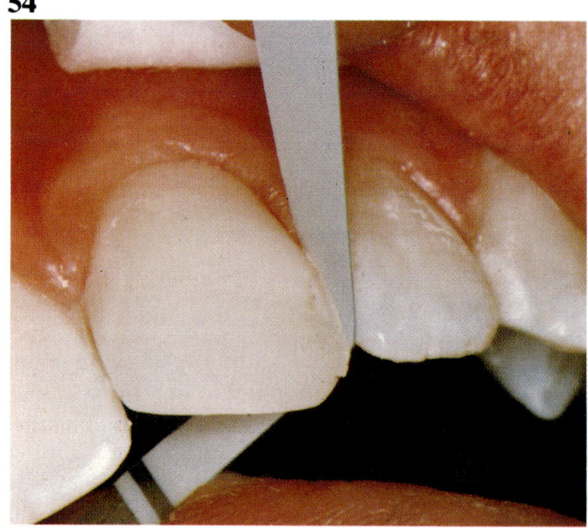

54 . . . a Soflex[R] polishing strip . . .

55

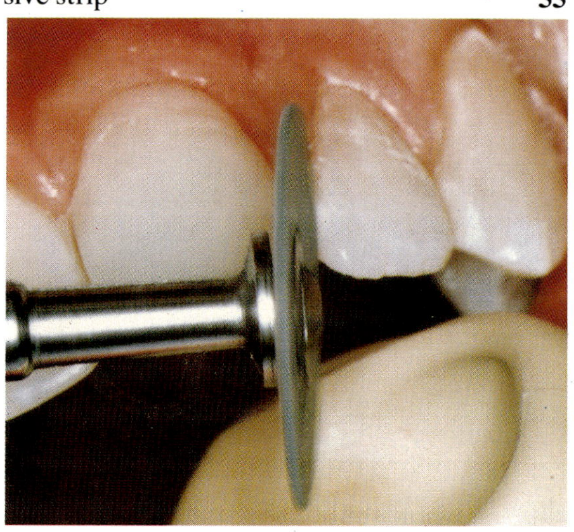

55 . . . or a Soflex[R] disc.

56

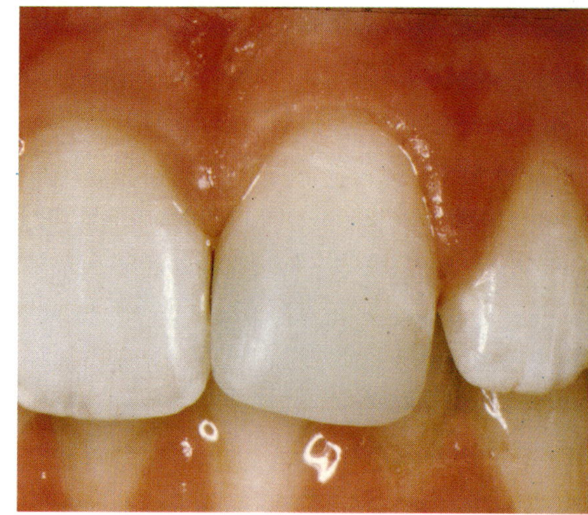

56 The final restoration.

Treatment of diastema

The method described above for restoring fractured incisors can be used to bond composite directly onto normal enamel in order to reduce a diastema.

57

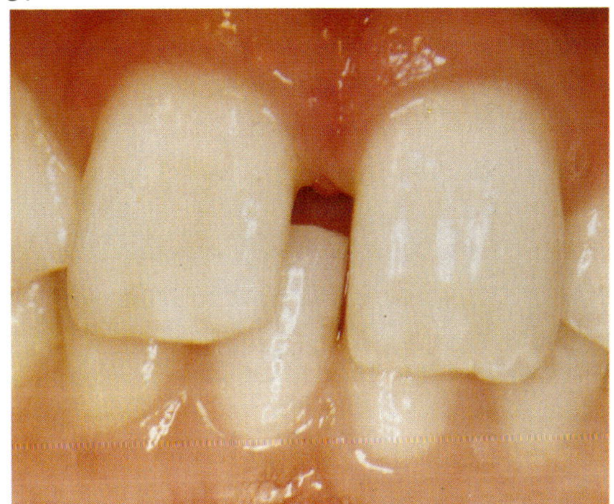

57 Diastema (3.5mm) between the upper central incisors.

58

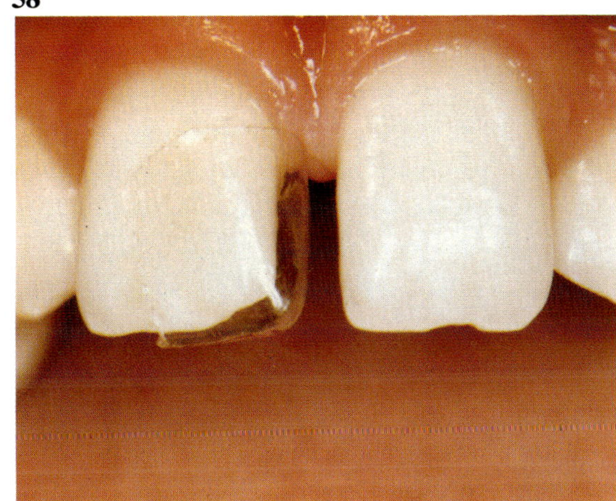

58 A suitable matrix is cut from a crown former.

59

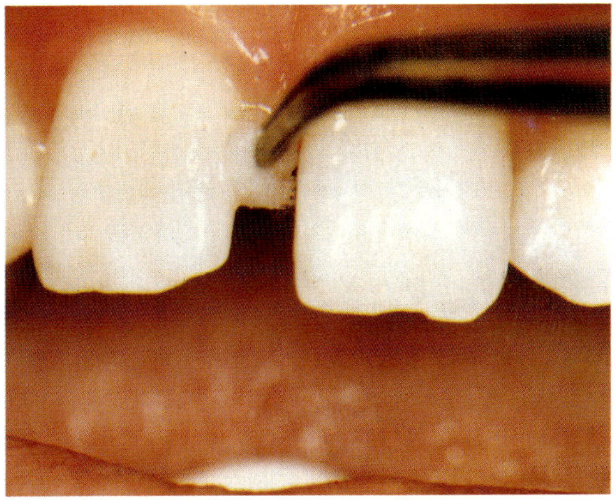

59 The tooth is etched for 60 seconds . . .

60

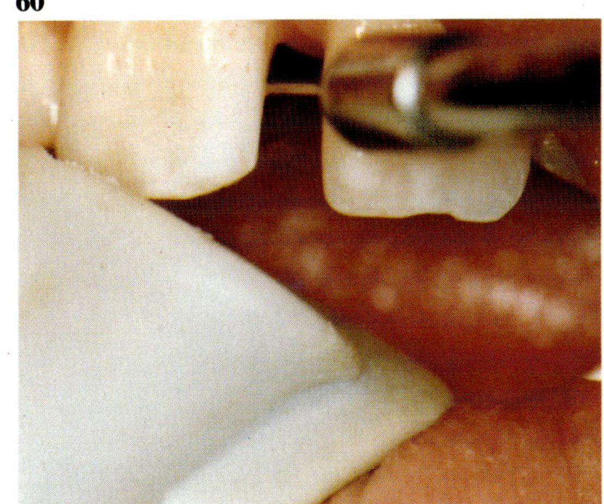

60 . . . washed for 10 seconds . . .

61

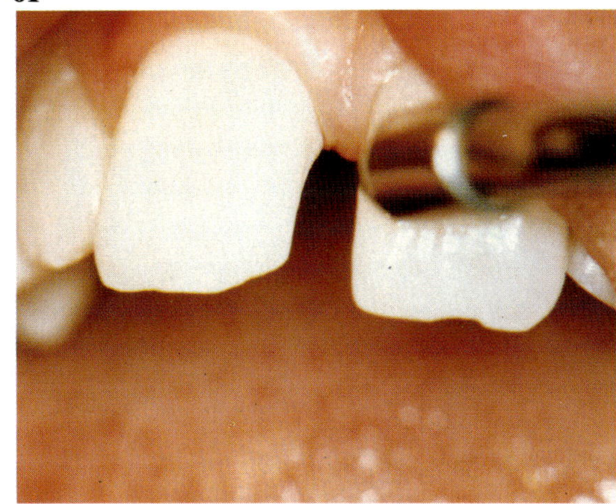

61 . . . and dried for 30 seconds.

62

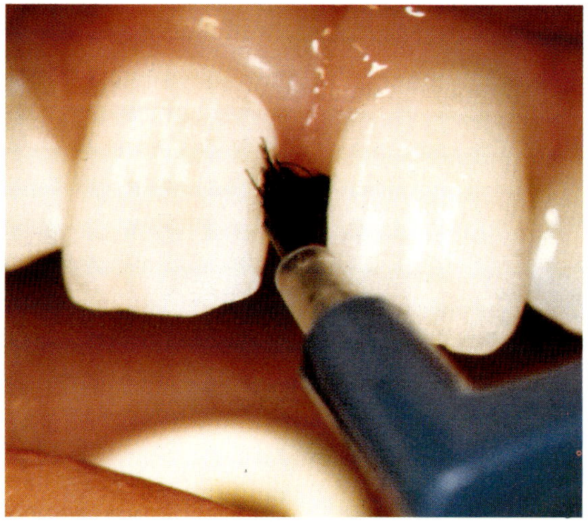

62 A bonding agent is then applied to the mesial surface with a brush.

63

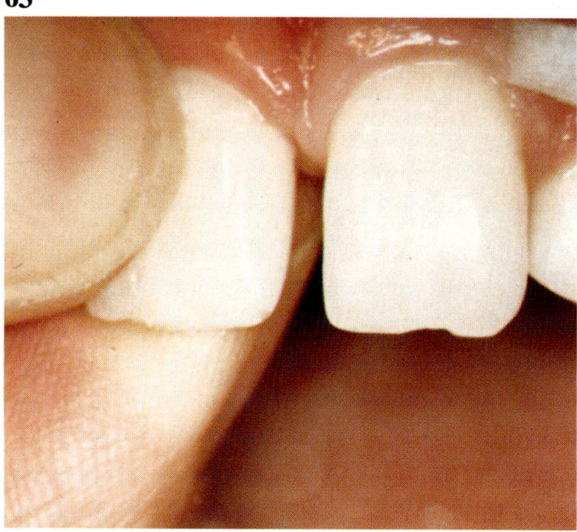

63 The matrix is filled with composite of the appropriate shade and applied to the tooth surface.

64

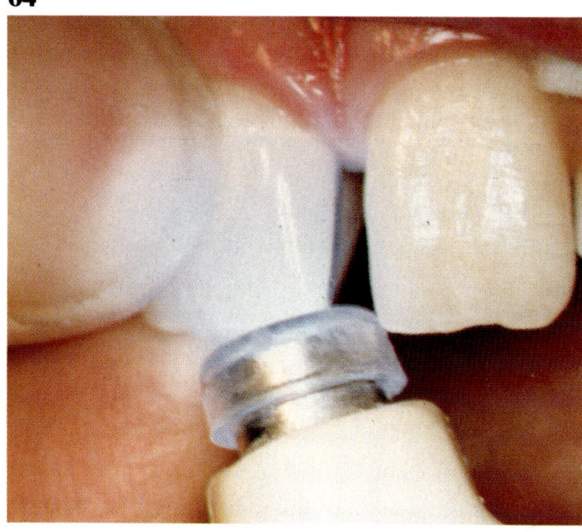

64 When the operator is satisfied with the position of the matrix the composite is cured with the light source.

65

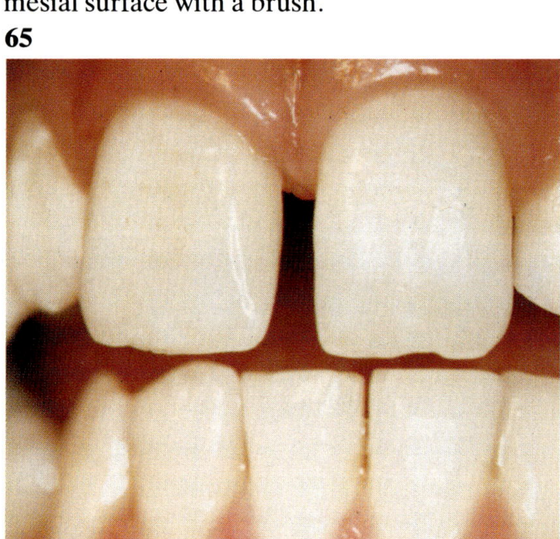

65 The finished result on the right central incisor.

66

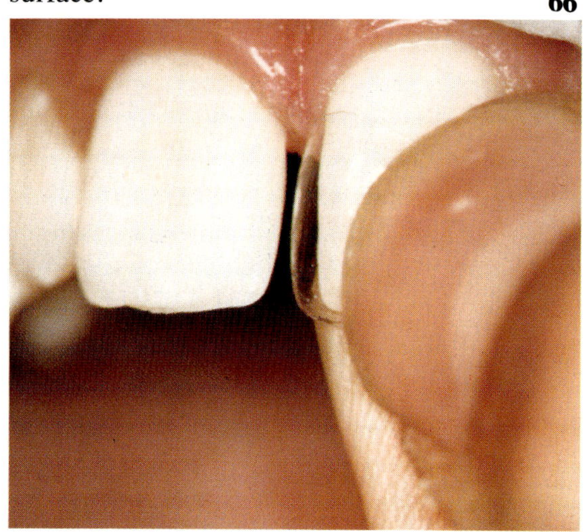

66 The same process, starting with a closely fitting matrix, is carried out on the left incisor.

67

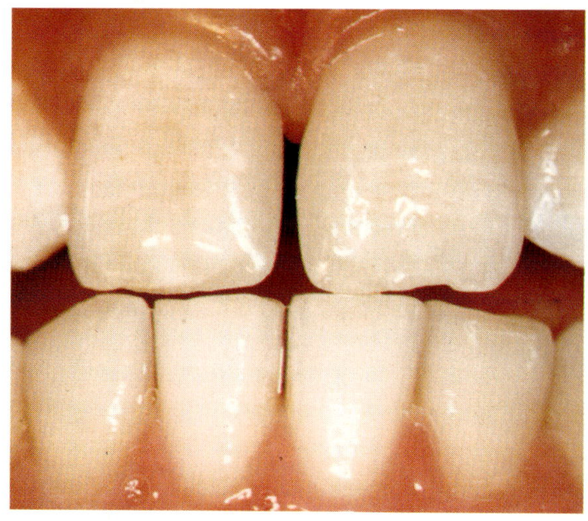

67 The final result – the diastema has now been reduced from 3.5mm to 0.5mm.

Construction of temporary crowns

The principles involved in restoring a fractured incisor or closing a diastema can also be extended to constructing a temporary crown; for example, to convert a lateral incisor into a central incisor, or to change a peg lateral incisor into a normal size lateral incisor. This can be particularly helpful as a temporary or semi-permanent measure in the developing dentition where the size of the pulp chamber would preclude the placing of porcelain crowns, which require cutting into the tooth. Either chemically-cured or light-sensitive composite material can be used.

68

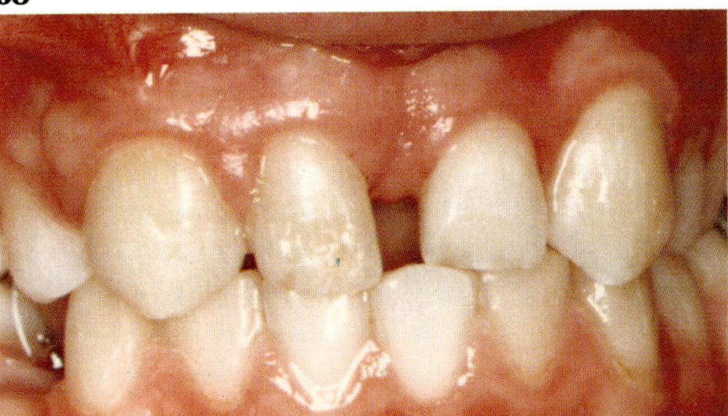

68 The upper central incisors in this patient were impacted because of the presence of supernumerary teeth. Even after the supernumerary teeth were removed the central incisors did not erupt, and had to be removed surgically.

69

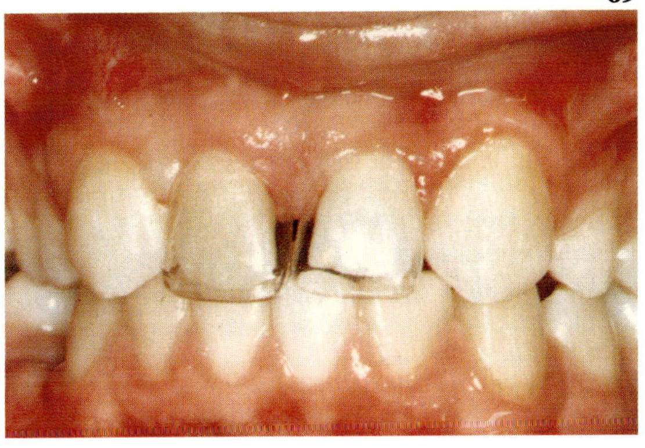

69 Crown formers are trimmed so that they fit tightly at the gingival margin but increase the size of the crown.

70

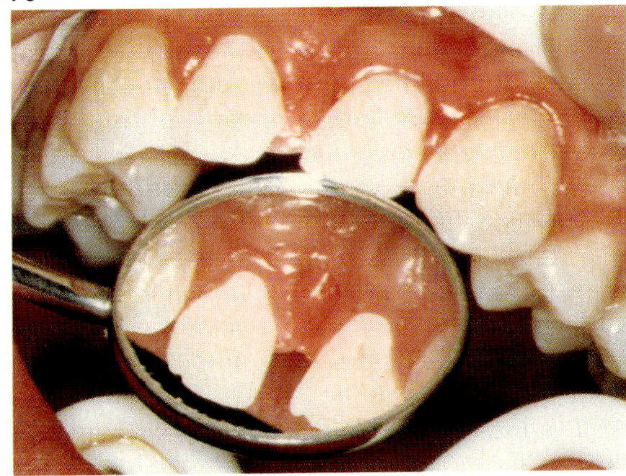

70 The whole of the crown, labial, palatal, mesial and distal is etched and then washed and dried. All surfaces of the tooth should now have a 'frosty' appearance.

71

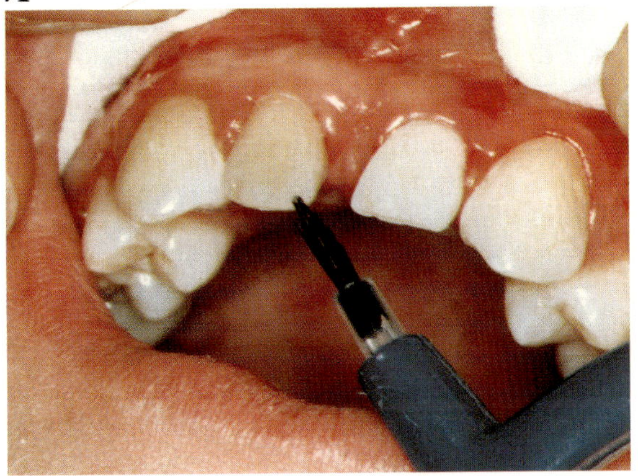

71 A bonding agent is applied to the tooth surface.

72

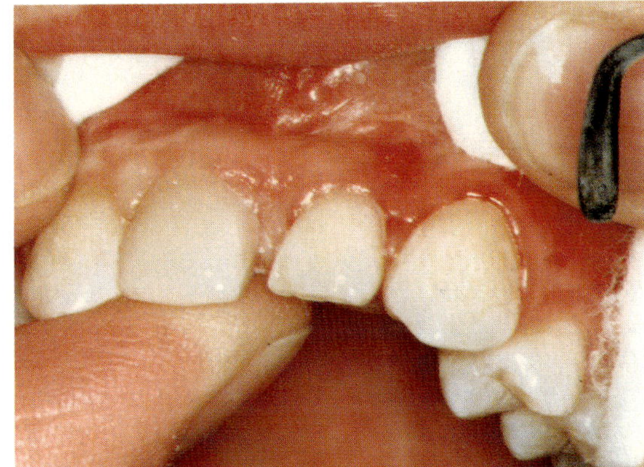

72 The crown former is filled with the composite resin (in this case a chemically cured microfil composite); it is placed on the upper right central incisor, the excess is removed and the crown is held in place for 5 minutes.

73

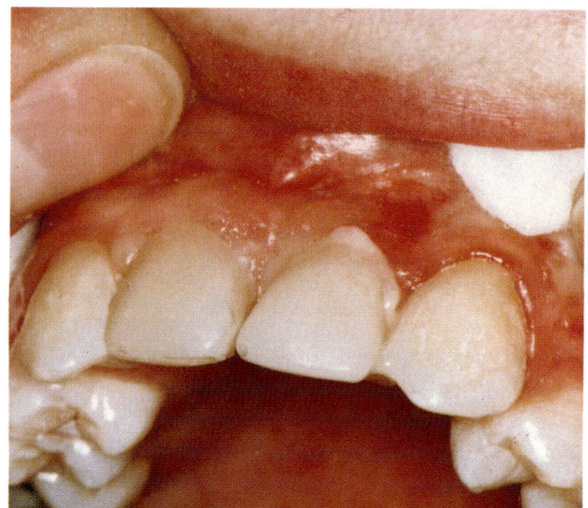

73 A similar procedure is carried out on the upper left incisor.

74

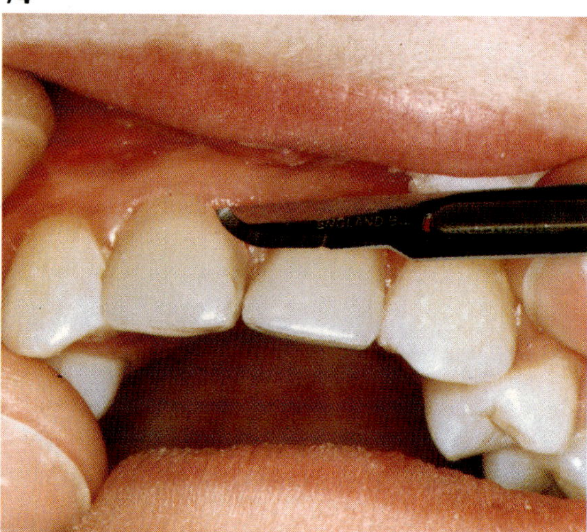

74 When the composite has set, the crown formers are removed with a scalpel.

75

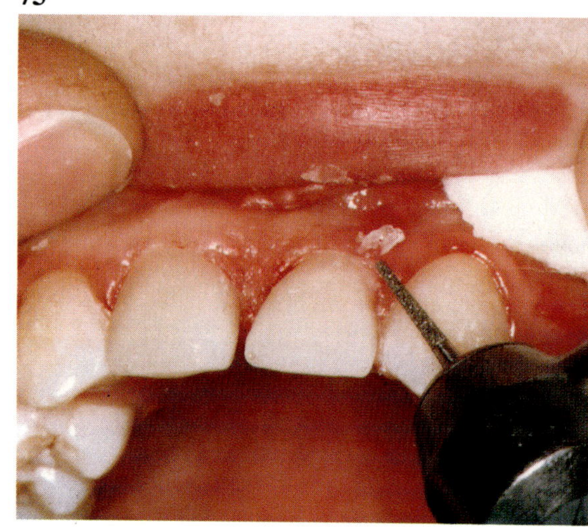

75 **Any excess composite is removed** with a fine tapered diamond bur.

76

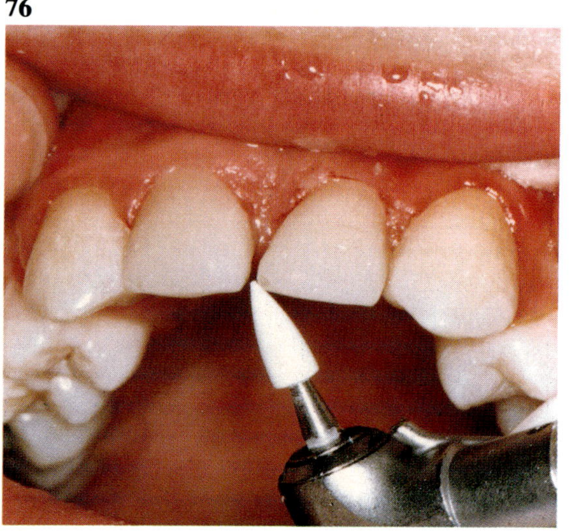

76 Final trimming can be carried out with a stone.

77

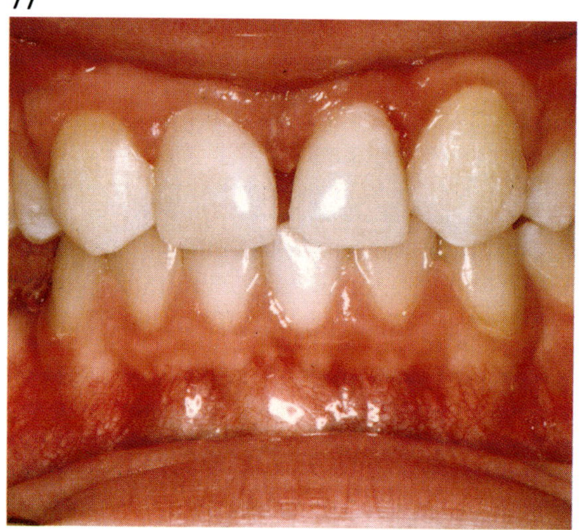

77 The final result from the labial aspect . . .

78

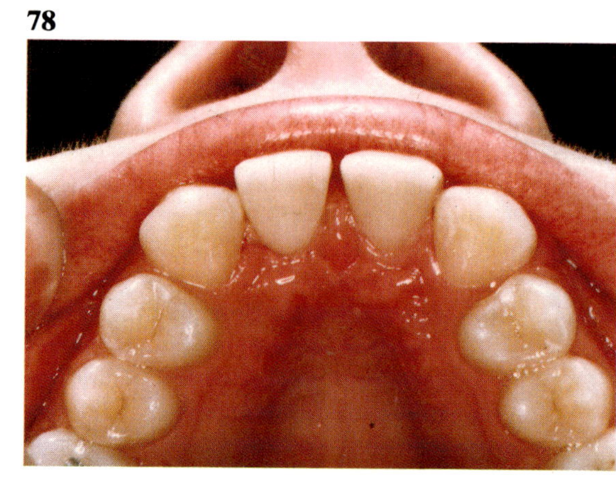

78 . . . and from the palatal aspect.

79

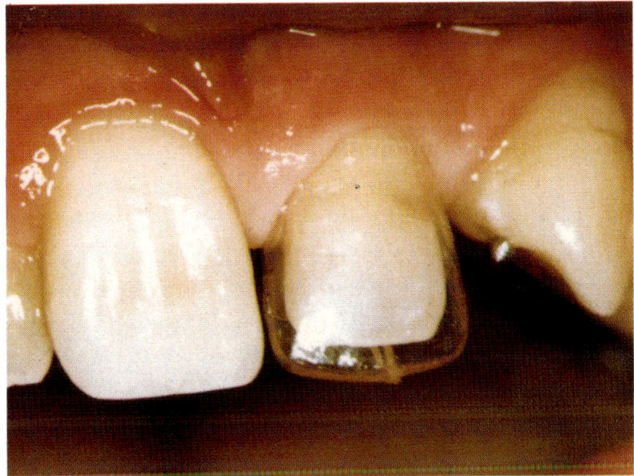

79 A similar technique employing a light sensitive material, can be used, for example, to convert an upper lateral incisor to a central incisor. A crown former is adapted to fit tightly at the gingival margin.

80

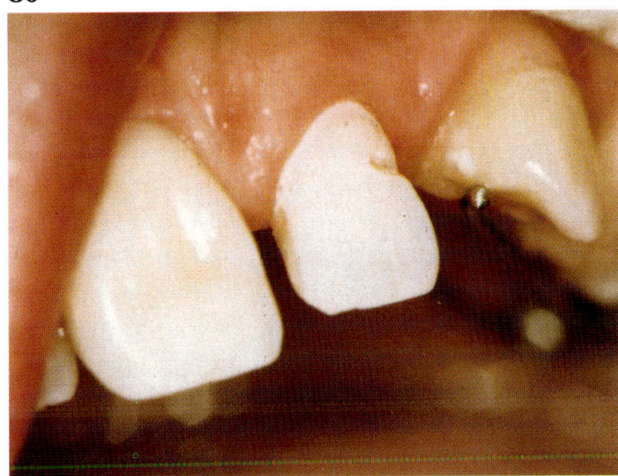

80 The tooth is etched, washed and dried to achieve a 'frosty' appearance.

81

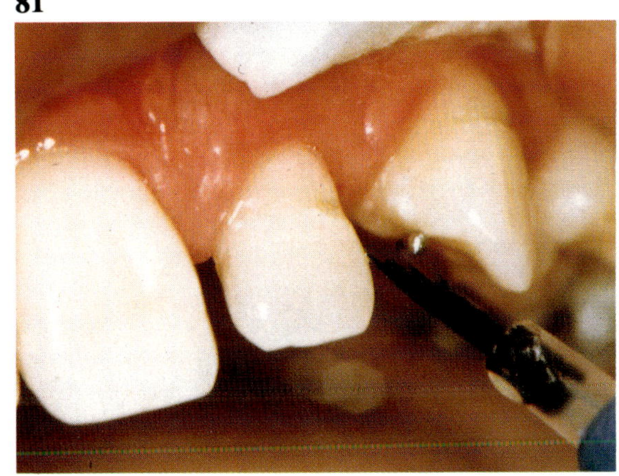

81 The bonding agent is applied with a brush.

82

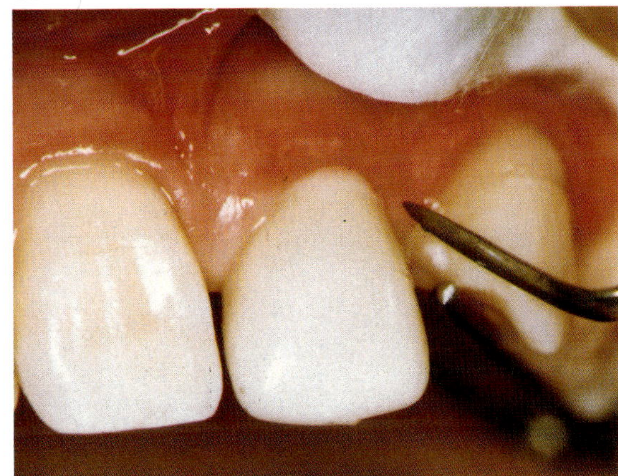

82 The crown former is filled with light sensitive composite resin of the appropriate shade and applied to the tooth. Time is available to trim any excess from the gingival margin.

83

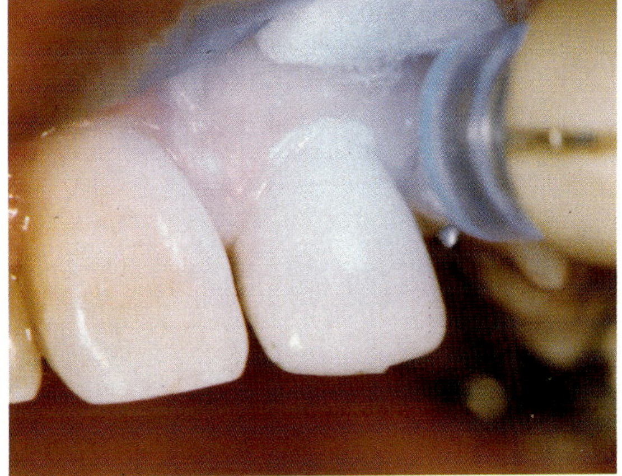

83 When all excess has been removed, the material is polymerised with the light. It will be necessary to shine the light both labially and palatally for at least 20 to 30 seconds because of the bulk of the material.

84

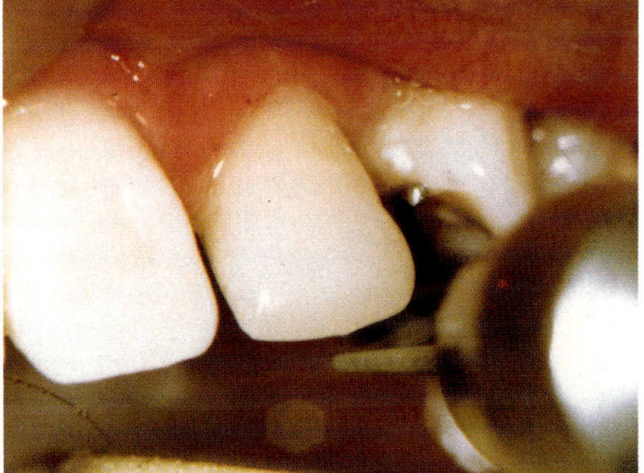

84 Adjustment of the incisal edge can be achieved with a fine tapered diamond bur.

Laminate veneers

Discoloured upper anterior teeth, particularly those stained by tetracyclines, are an extremely difficult clinical problem. On the one hand the tooth structure is usually sound and free from decay and therefore from a clinical point of view it is difficult to cut into sound tissue and risk damaging the pulp. On the other hand, from the patient's view the teeth are discoloured and unsightly. In the past the usual line of treatment was to delay treatment until the patient reached 16 to 18 years of age, when porcelain jacket crowns could be provided. However, the development of the acid etch technique enables plastic veneers to be bonded to the labial enamel surface, so improving the appearance.

A number of developments in the laminate veneer technique have taken place in the last few years. Initially, the pre-formed veneers were trimmed at the chair-side and a chemically cured composite resin was used to attach the veneer to the etched enamel surface. It was not always possible to adapt a pre-formed veneer very closely to some incisor teeth and an indirect technique was developed, whereby the veneers were trimmed on a model and then heat adapted to the labial surface in the laboratory. The use of a light-sensitive resin was introduced which gave the flexibility of 'command cure'. Greater time was available to place the veneers in the optimum position and any excess composite could be removed while it was still soft. When the clinician was satisfied with the position of the veneer the composite was then polymerised quickly with the light source.

85

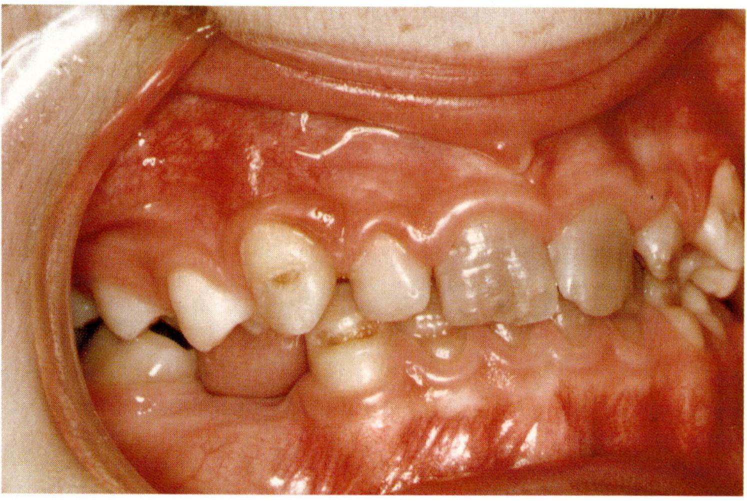

85 Badly stained central incisor teeth.

86

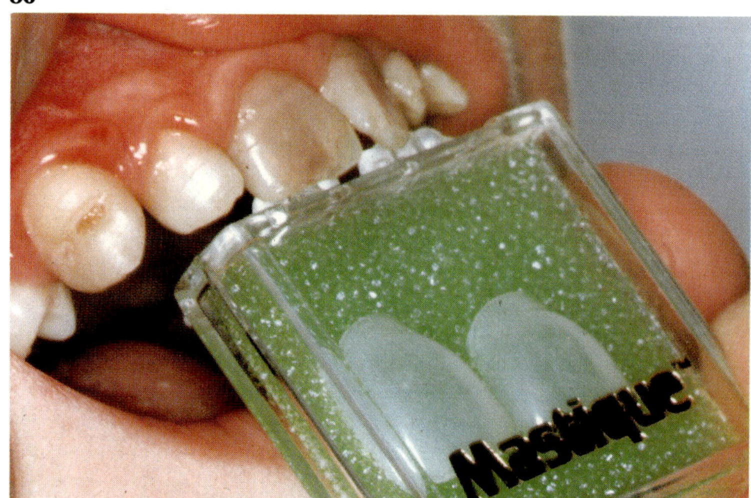

86 A pre-formed laminate veneer (Mastique[R]) is chosen which most closely approximates to the size of the tooth.

87

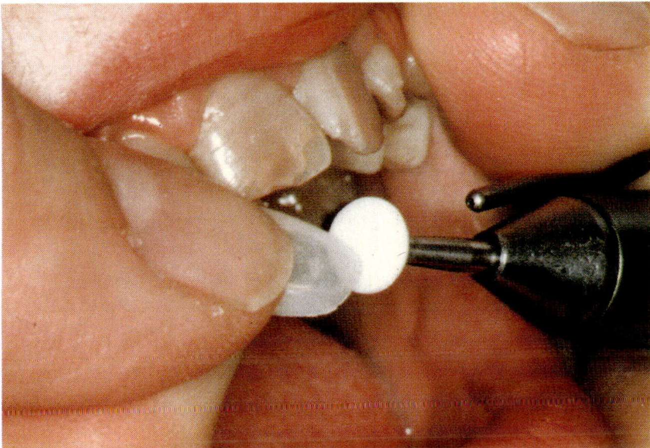

87 The veneer is trimmed and smoothed with a white stone . . .

88

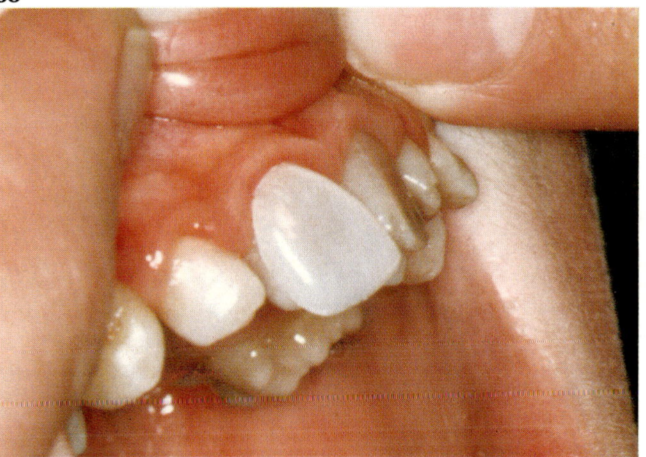

88 . . . so that it fits just into the gingival crevice. The length of the veneer is then reduced until it does not extend beyond the natural incisal edge.

89

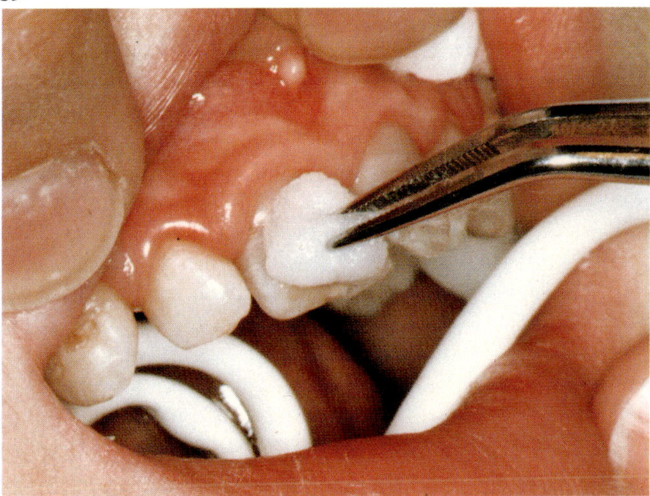

89 The labial surface is then etched, washed and dried in the normal way.

90

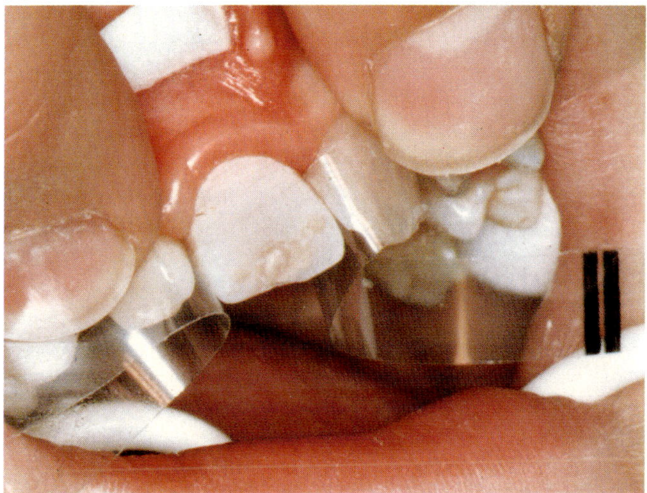

90 Celluloid strips are placed on the adjacent teeth. Note the 'frosty' appearance of the etched labial surface.

91

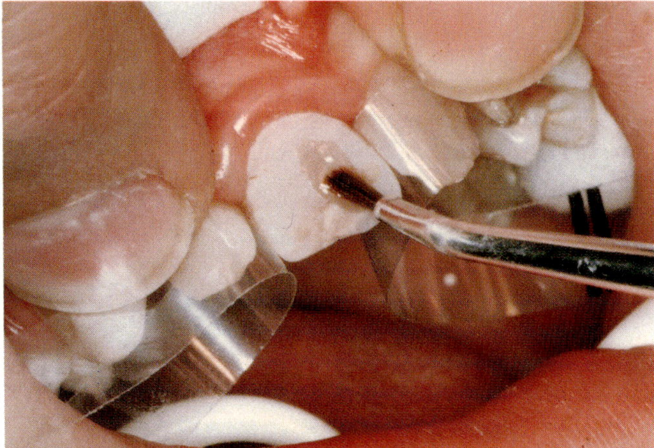

91 Bonding agent is painted on the etched surface.

92

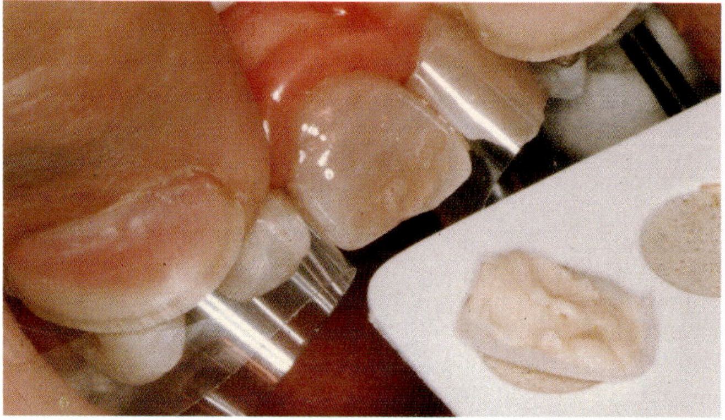

92 **The veneer,** which has been cleaned and primed for ten minutes with the agent provided, is then filled with composite of the appropriate shade and placed on the labial surface.

93

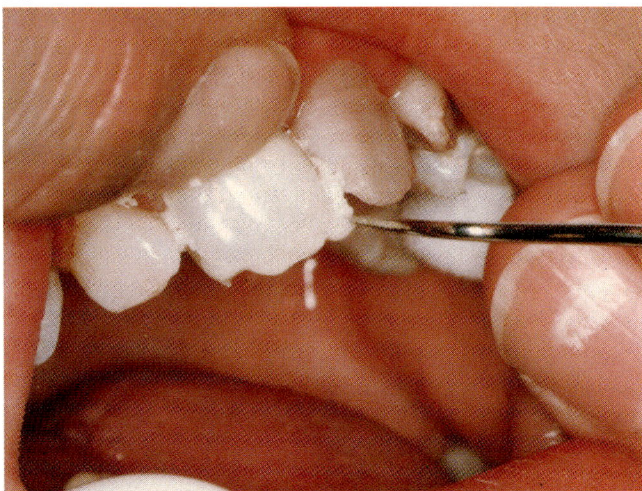

93 **Some excess material can be removed with a probe,** but the veneer must be held firmly in place for three minutes and then not touched for a further two minutes, to allow chemical polymerisation to take place.

94

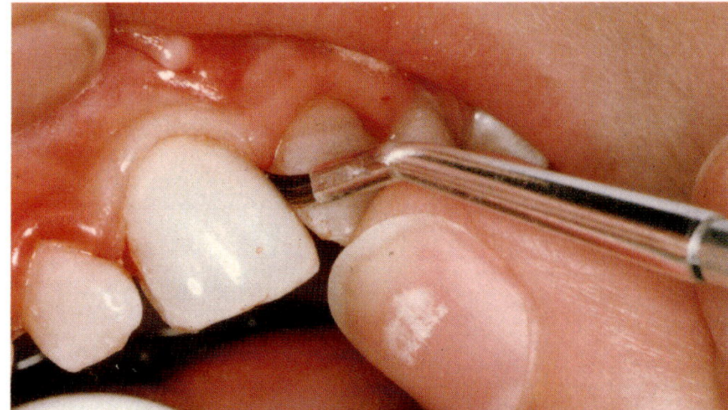

94 **After five minutes any remaining excess composite is removed** with sandpaper discs or a tapered diamond bur. The incisal edge should be trimmed so that the force of the occlusion is taken on the natural incisal edge, rather than on the veneer. Finally, the margins of the veneer are sealed with a further application of the bonding agent with a paintbrush.

One of the problems with this technique is that, unless the laminate is an extremely good fit, the tooth is made rather bulky in a labio-lingual direction. Another problem is that there is a danger of pressing too hard on the laminate veneer whilst waiting for the composite to polymerise, so introducing strains into the veneer-composite interface.

These problems can be reduced by ensuring a close-fitting veneer by preparing them on a model in the laboratory and heat treating the veneer to adapt it to the model. Furthermore, the polymerising time can be reduced by using the visible light curing composite, which enables the veneer to be positioned gently and then cured in 20 to 60 seconds.

95

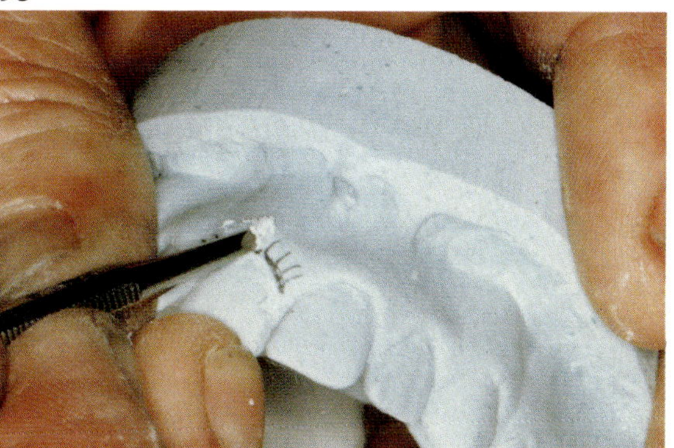

95 An impression of the upper arch was taken from which the plaster model shown was made. A chisel is used to remove a small amount of plaster at the gingival margin so that the veneer will fit below the gingival margin.

96

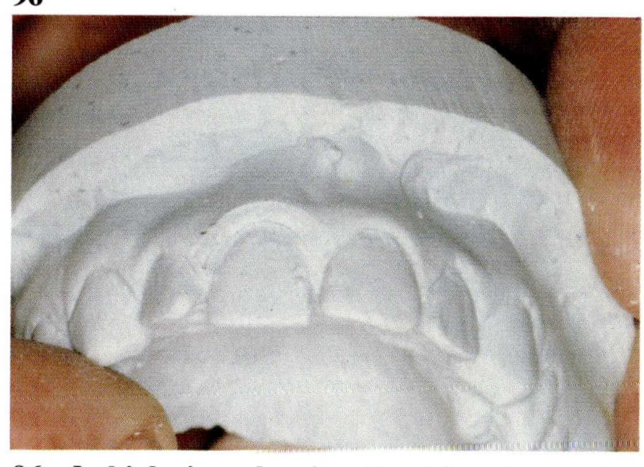

96 Labial view showing the trimming of the plaster around the gingival margin of the upper right central incisor.

97

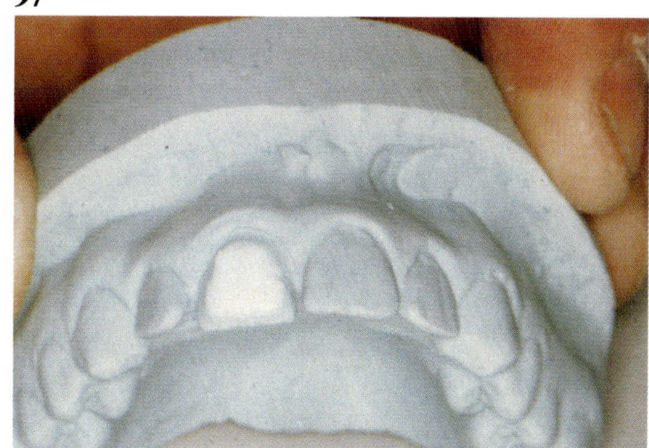

97 A latex compound is spread evenly over the middle of the labial surface to act as a 'spacer' for the composite resin which attaches the veneer to the tooth surface.

98

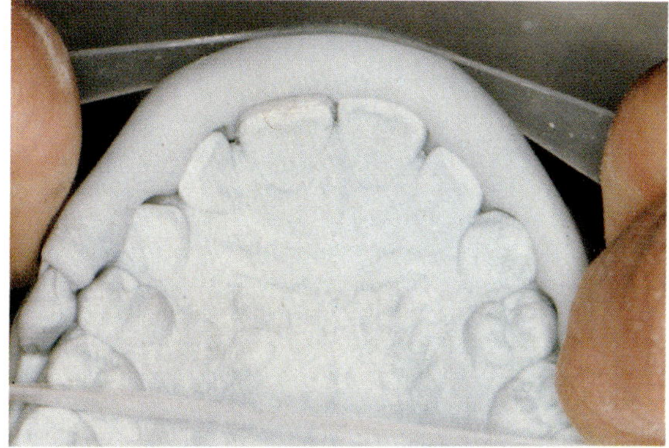

98 When all the veneers have been trimmed, silicone impression material is held firmly in place against the veneers, with an elastic band. The model is then placed in a machine which applies heat and pressure so that the veneers are softened and adapted more closely to the labial surface of the teeth.

99

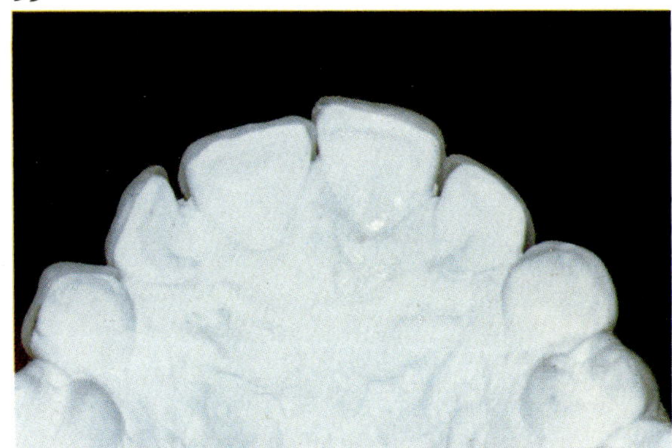

99 The heat adapted veneers closely adapted to the model.

100

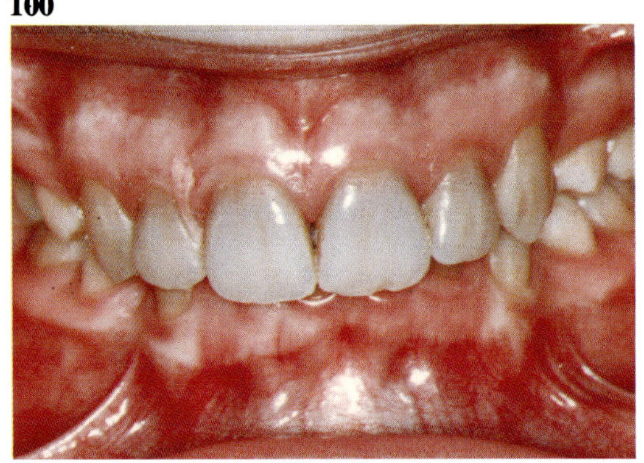

100 The indirect method of preparing laminate veneers, together with the use of the Prisma light to cure the composite, was used on the following patient with tetracycline staining.

101

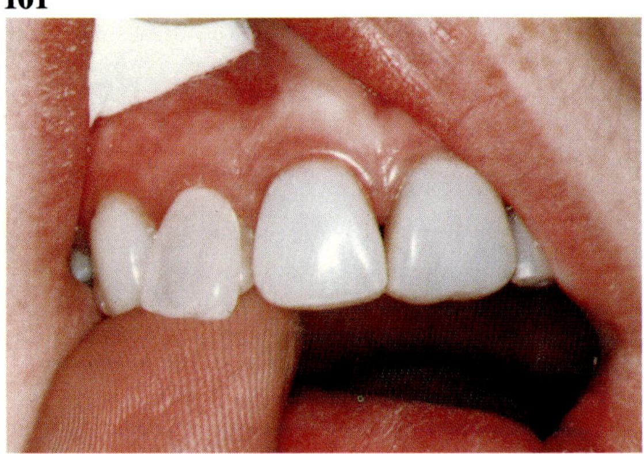

101 The prepared veneer is checked on the labial surface of the upper right lateral incisor.

102

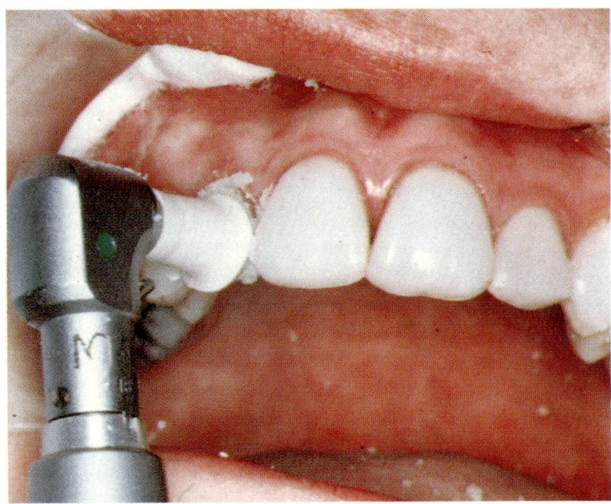

102 The tooth is then cleaned with pumice, washed and dried.

103

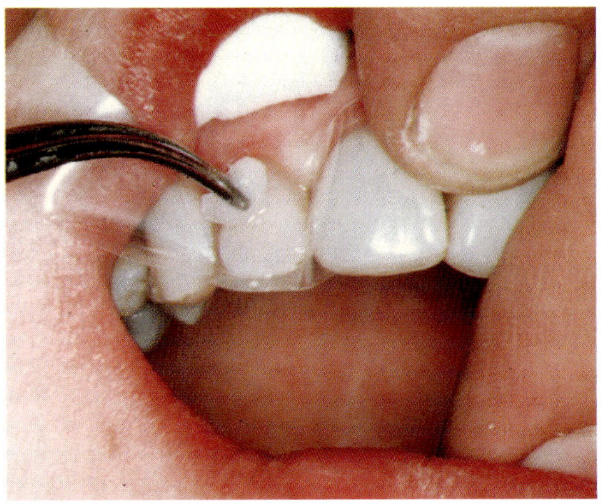

103 Celluloid strips are placed in the interstitial areas on either side of the tooth, which is then etched . . .

104

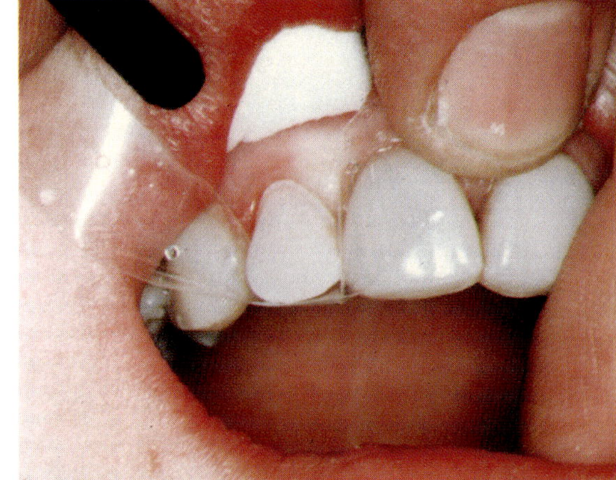

104 . . . washed and dried to achieve the necessary 'frosty' appearance.

105

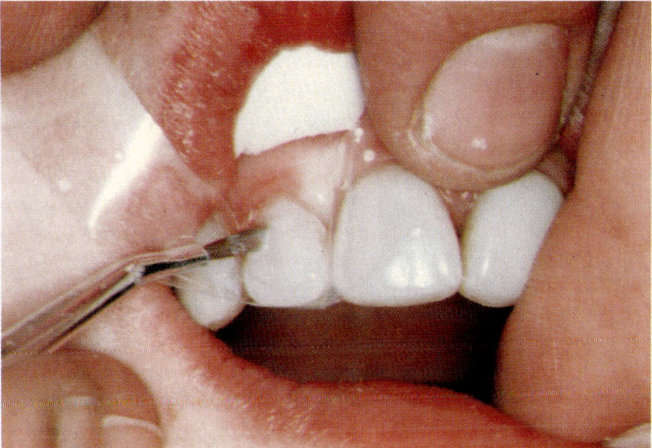

105 The opaquer being applied to the labial surface to prevent the darkness of the tooth showing through the composite.

106

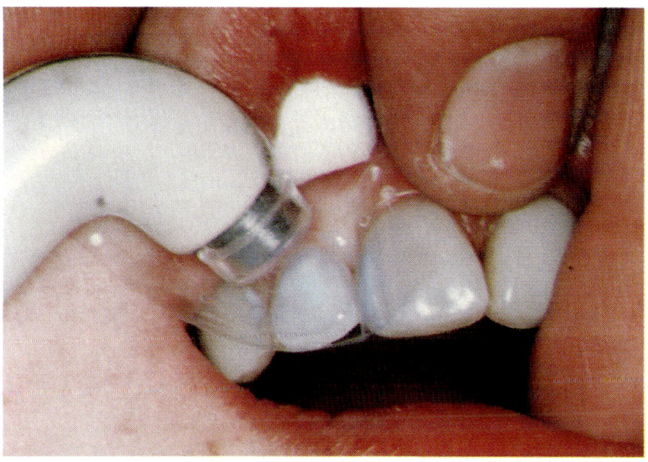

106 Curing the opaquer for 10 seconds.

107

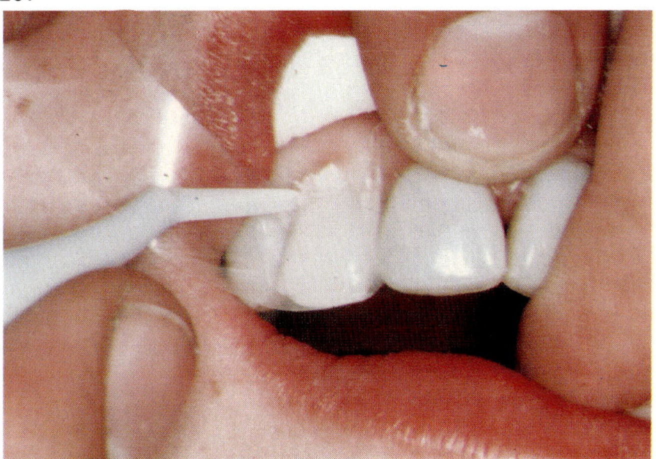

107 The veneer, coated with composite, is placed on the labial surface and any excess composite is removed with a plastic instrument.

108

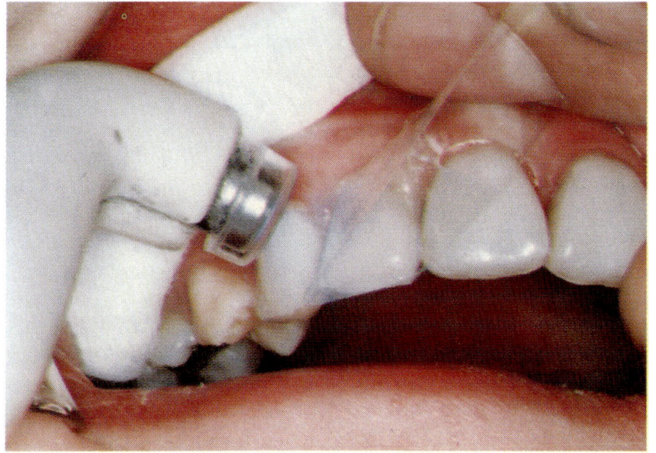

108 When the operator is satisfied with the position of the veneer, the composite is cured with the light for 50 to 60 seconds.

109

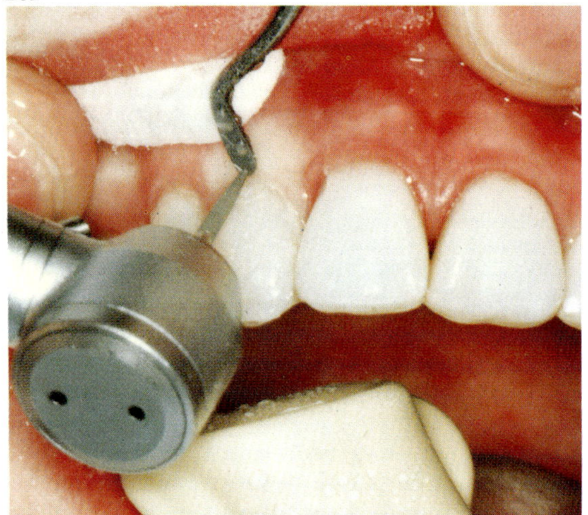

110

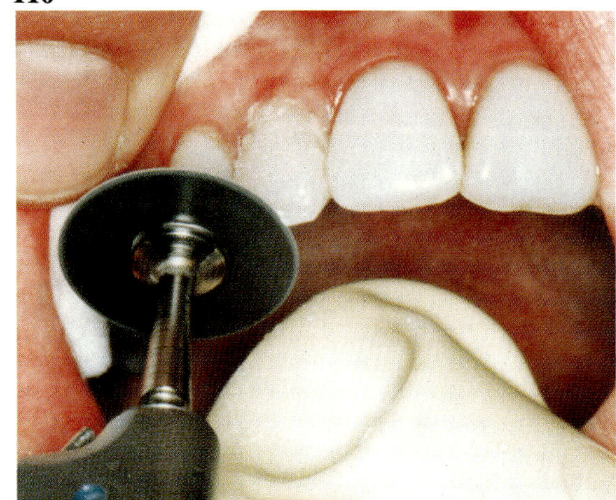

111

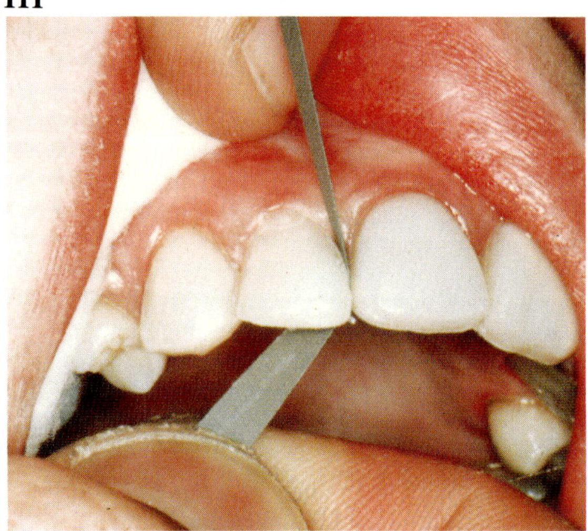

109 Final trimming can be carried out with a diamond composite finishing bur . . .

110 . . . a flexible abrasive disc (Soflex^{R}) and . . .

111 . . . an abrasive strip (Soflex^{R}).

112

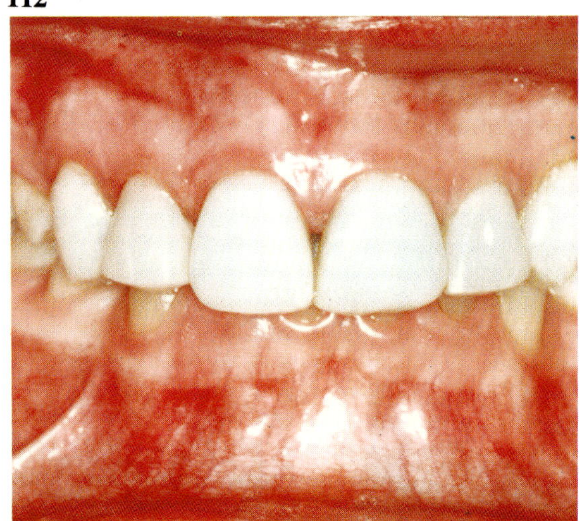

112 The final appearance – labial view.

113

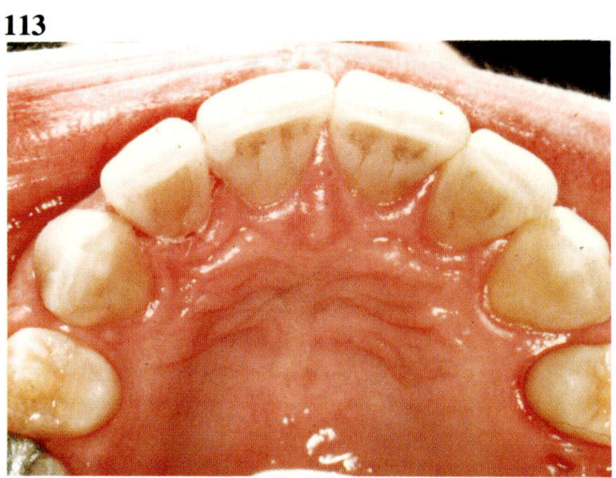

113 Palatal view, showing the slight increase in the bulk of the tooth.

Splinting subluxated and luxated teeth

Front teeth, particularly upper incisor teeth, are frequently damaged by injuries in childhood. From the first faltering steps in infancy to involvement in 'contact' sports, teeth are in the 'front line'. The treatment of fractured incisors has been considered in an earlier chapter. Sometimes, rather than snap off a piece of the crown, the force of the injury loosens the whole tooth so that it is either loosened (subluxated) or displaced (luxated).

The best treatment for luxated teeth is to reduce the displacement by repositioning them as quickly and gently as possible. Both subluxated and luxated teeth are then held in place with a splint. In the past a cast metal or acrylic splint was made. This required an impression to be taken of the arch involved, which in itself caused further damage to the traumatised site by the pressure involved when removing the impression. The acid etch technique enables a tooth to be splinted gently in the correct position with virtually no disturbance to the injured areas.

114

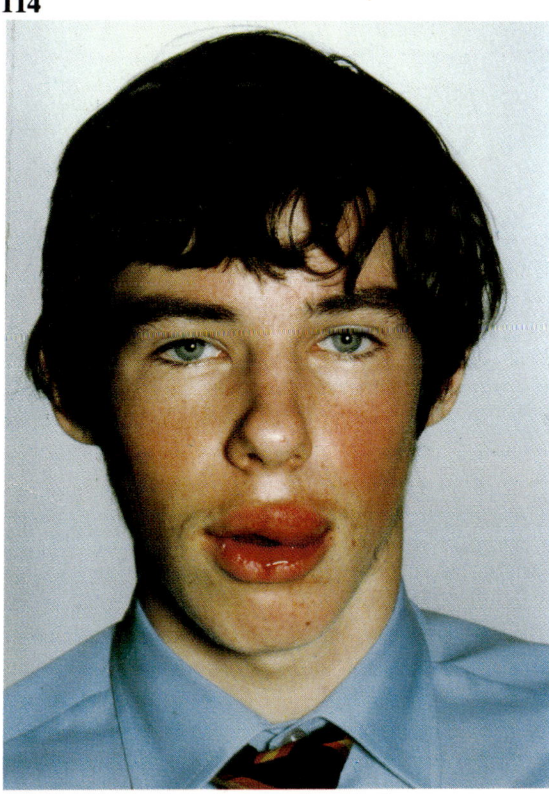

114 A boy aged 15 years who had been hit in the face with a cricket ball.

115

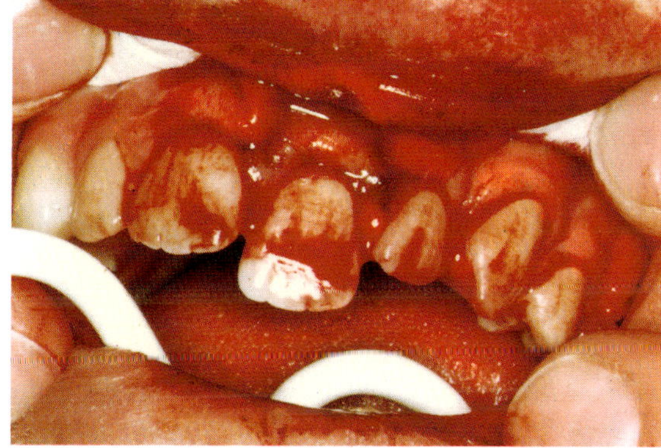

115 Intra-oral view, showing that the upper left central incisor had been partly extruded from its socket.

116

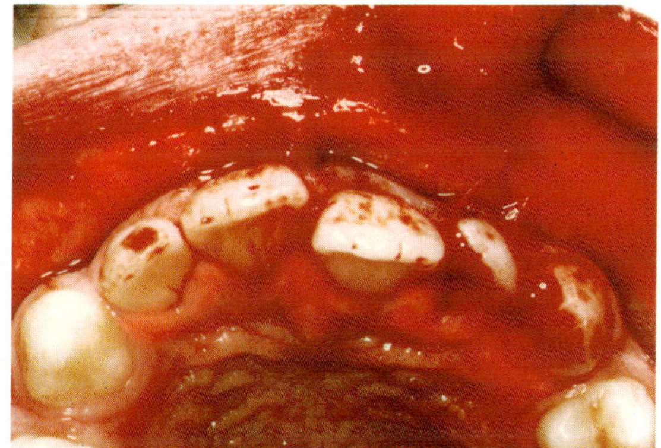

116 Palatal view, showing that the left central incisor had also been pushed backwards.

117

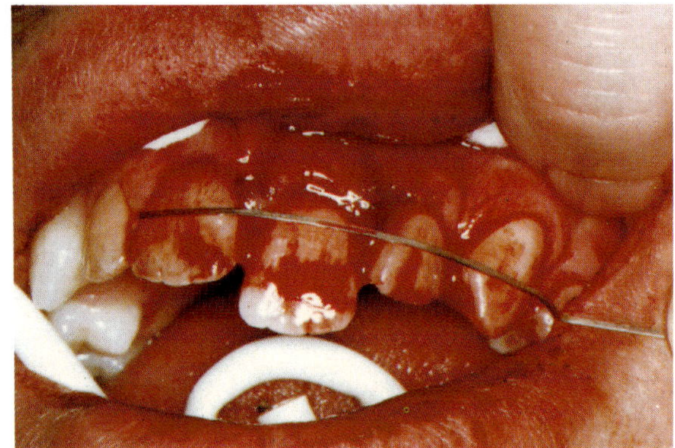

117 A piece of orthodontic wire is adapted to fit over the labial surface of the misplaced tooth and the adjacent teeth.

118

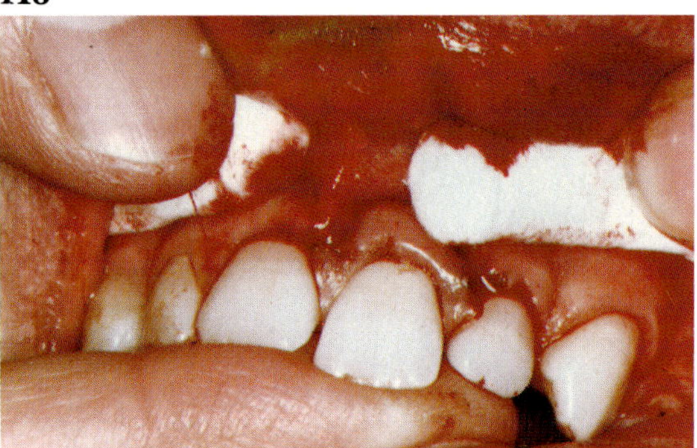

118 The tooth is manipulated gently back into position and maintained there with finger pressure.

119

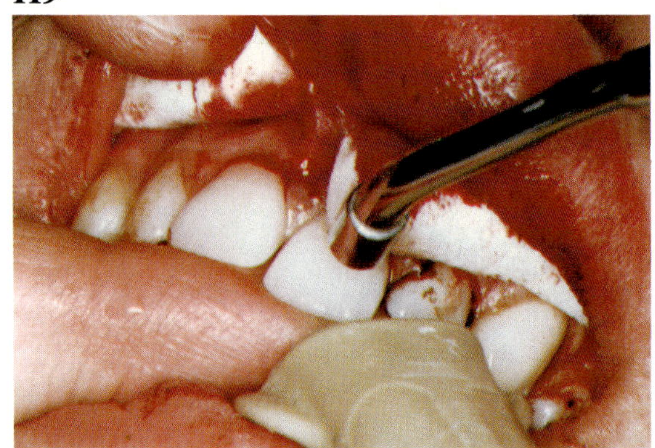

119 The area is isolated with cottonwool rolls and the labial surfaces of the affected tooth, and one or two teeth on either side of it, are washed and dried.

120

120 These surfaces are then etched, washed and dried in the normal way, to achieve a 'frosty' appearance.

121

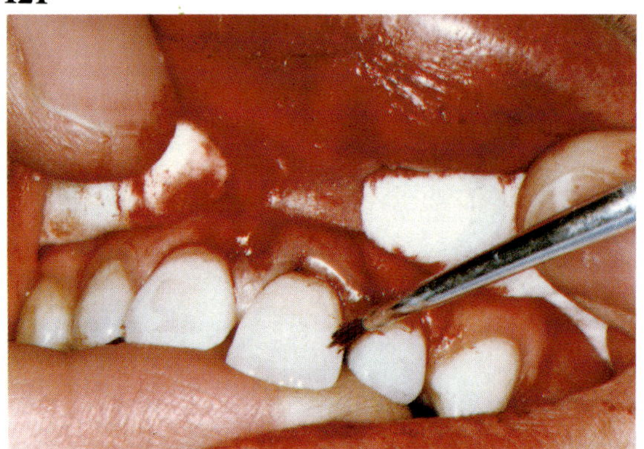

121 A small amount of light-sensitive composite is then placed on the acid etched area of each tooth . . .

122

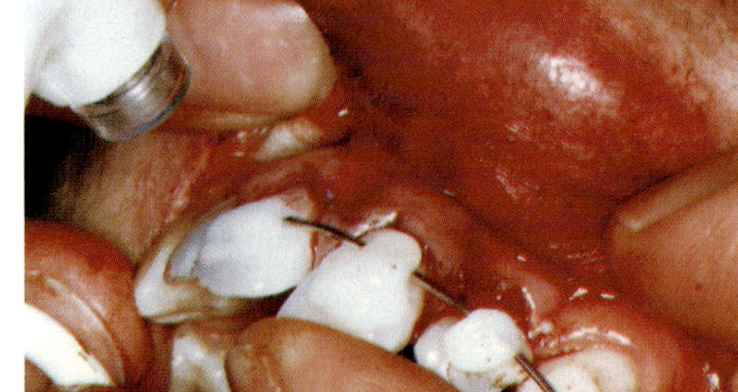

122 . . . the orthodontic wire is placed in position and more composite is added to hold the wire in the correct position. The composite is then cured with the light system.

123

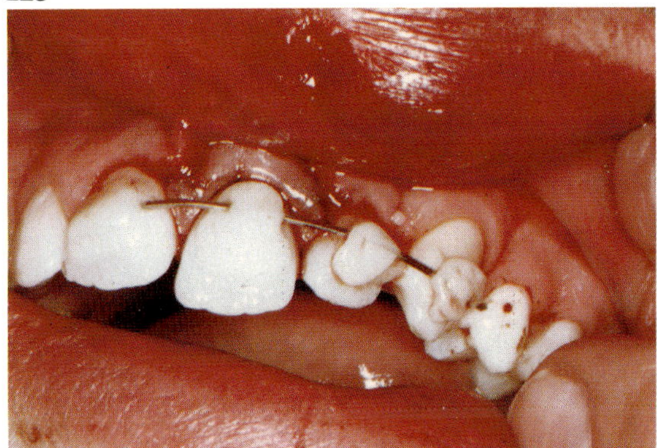

123 The splint in position. Note that, in spite of maintaining finger pressure on the incisal edge of the traumatised tooth during all the previous procedures, the incisal edge of the upper left central incisor is slightly below that of the right central incisor. However, it was not possible to seat the loose tooth any further into its socket.

124

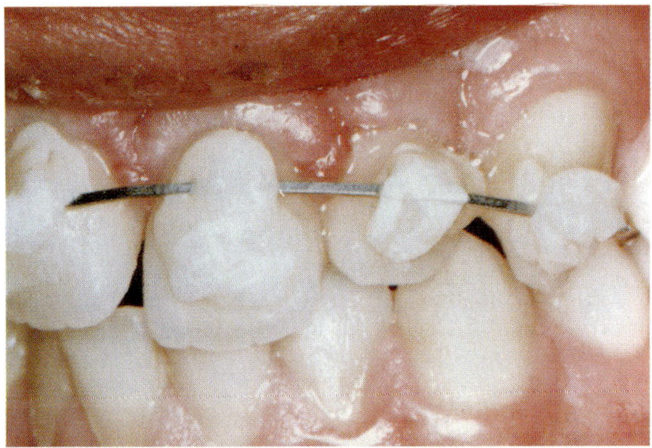

124 The condition of the splint one month later, when it was removed.

126

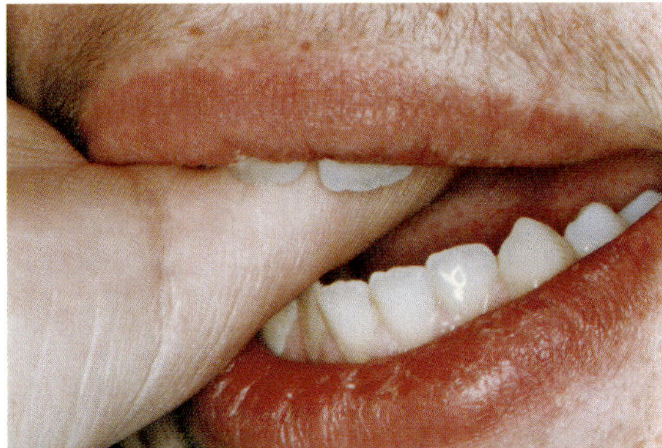

126 The reason for the difference in the level of the incisal edges of the two central incisors was revealed – the patient still sucked his right thumb!

125

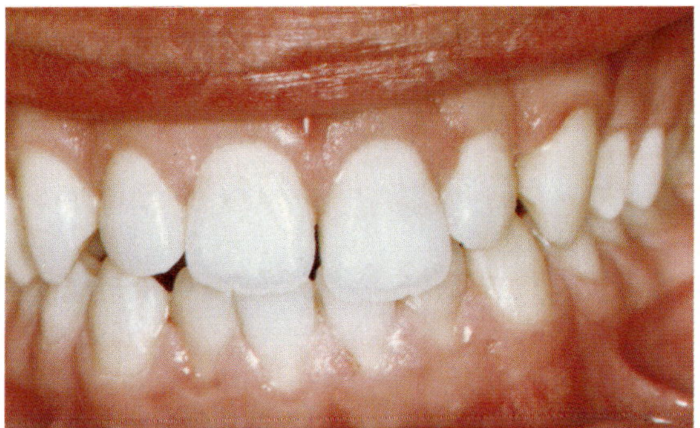

125 The teeth were polished, and the affected tooth was of good colour and in an acceptable position.

127

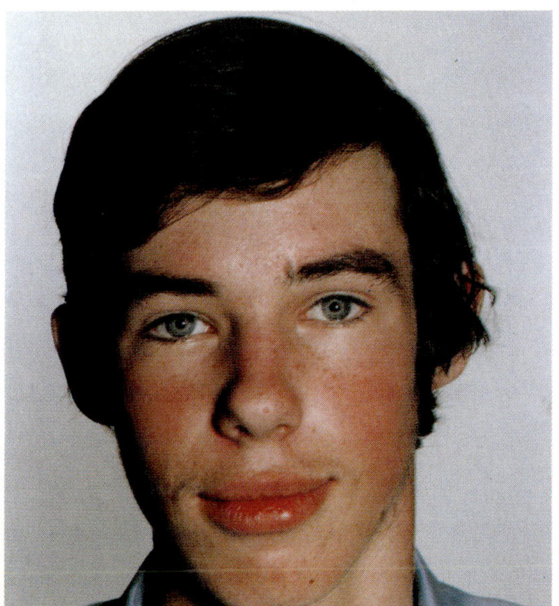

127 Although the superficial facial injuries healed quickly, the injury to the tooth was such that death of the pulp occurred, and the tooth was root-filled.

Acid etch retained bridges

Whenever an incisor tooth is luxated or avulsed the treatment of choice is to reposition it immediately. If this does not happen, and the tooth is lost, the only treatment then available is to provide a denture, at least in the short or medium term. With the advent of the acid etch technique, a simple impression of the affected arch is taken and a 'Rochette' Bridge constructed, with a pontic and two butterfly extensions which have been adapted to fit closely to the palatal surfaces of the abutment teeth. The wings of the bridge have 3 to 5 holes through which the composite flows and retains the bridge in position.

128

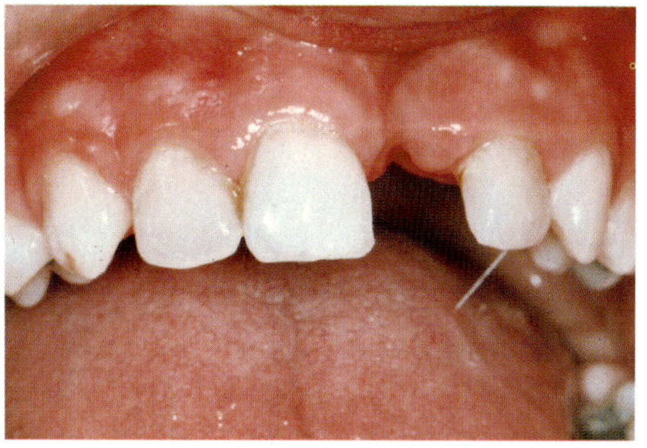

128 A child aged 12 years who had knocked out her upper left central incisor three years previously following an accident while riding her bicycle.

129

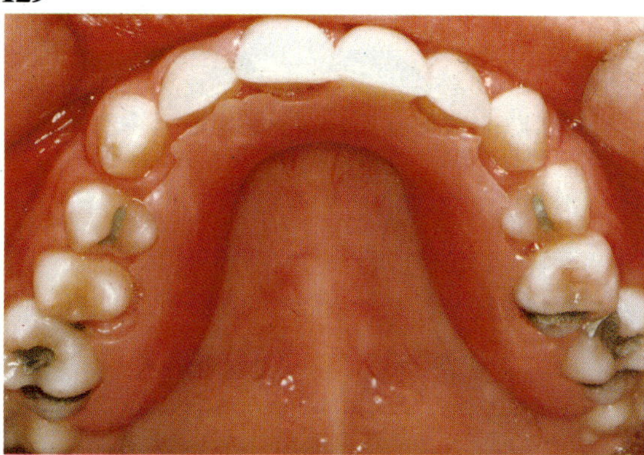

129 A palatal view of the denture replacing the missing incisor, showing the 'gum-stripping' design of the denture.

130

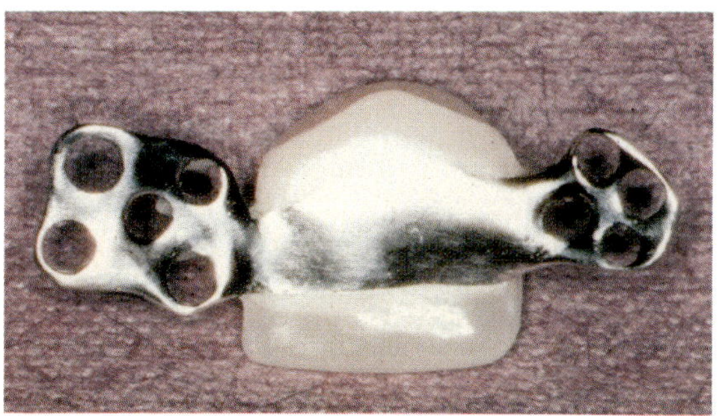

130 Palatal view of a 'Rochette' Bridge, showing the pontic and two butterfly extensions which have been constructed to fit closely to the palatal surfaces of the abutment teeth.

131

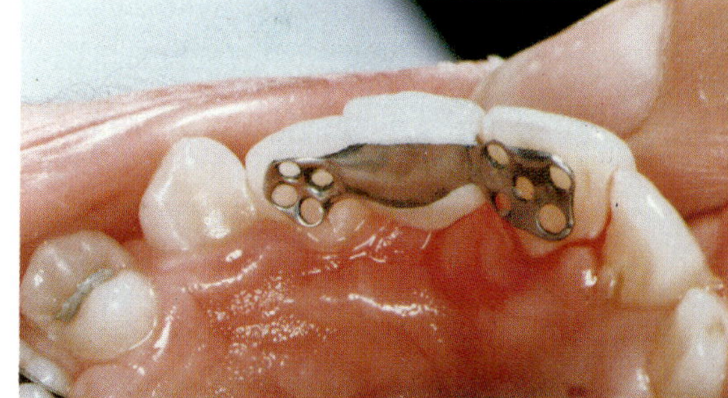

131 Palatal view showing the bridge in position, before cementation.

132

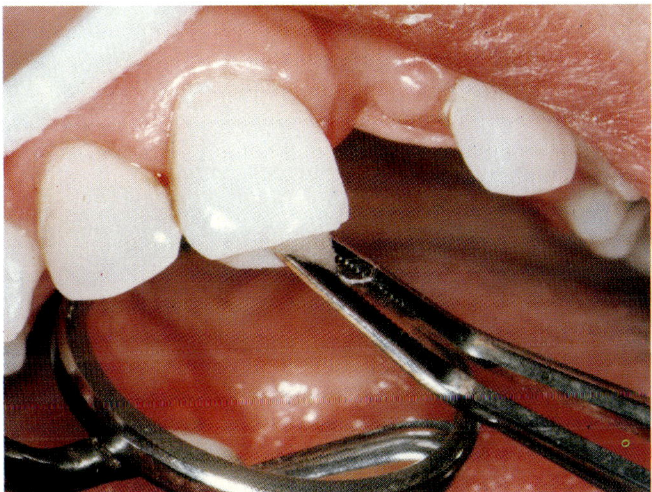

132 Following a thorough prophylaxis the palatal surfaces of the abutment teeth are etched for 60 seconds . . .

133

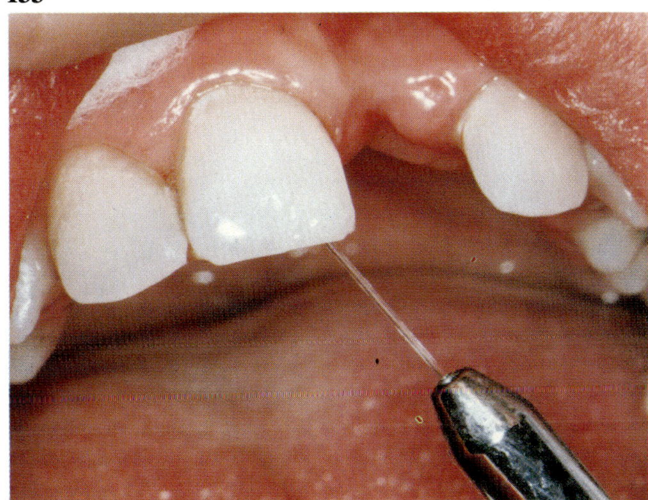

133 . . . washed for 30 seconds . . .

134

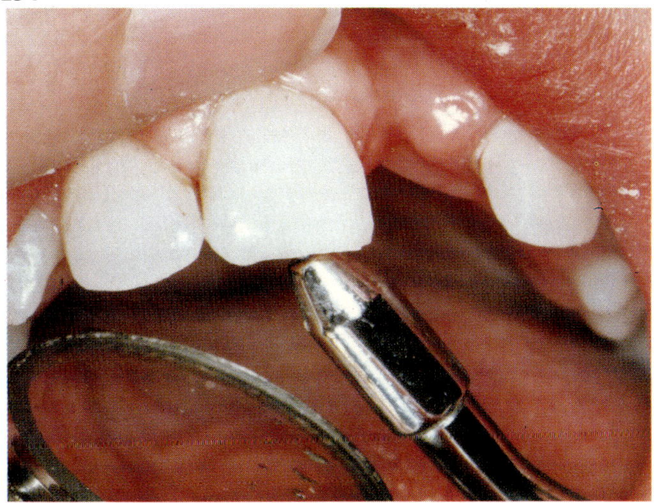

134 . . . and dried thoroughly . . .

135

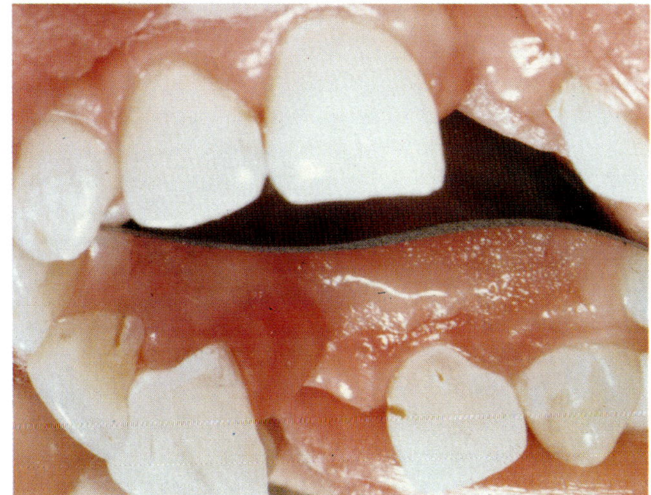

135 . . . to achieve the usual 'frosty' appearance.

136

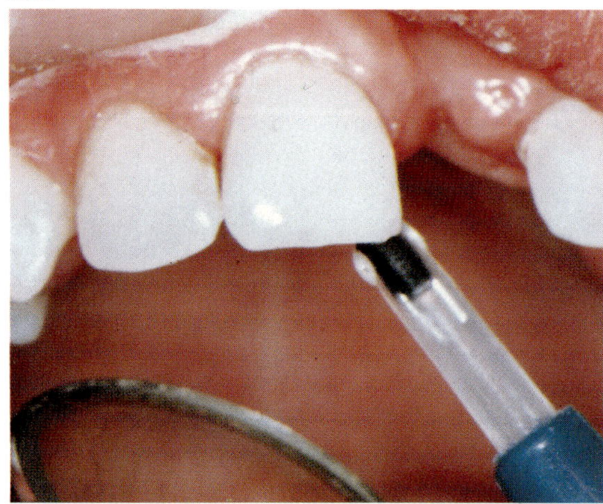

136 The area is isolated with cottonwool rolls and bonding agent is then applied to the palatal surfaces of the abutment teeth.

137

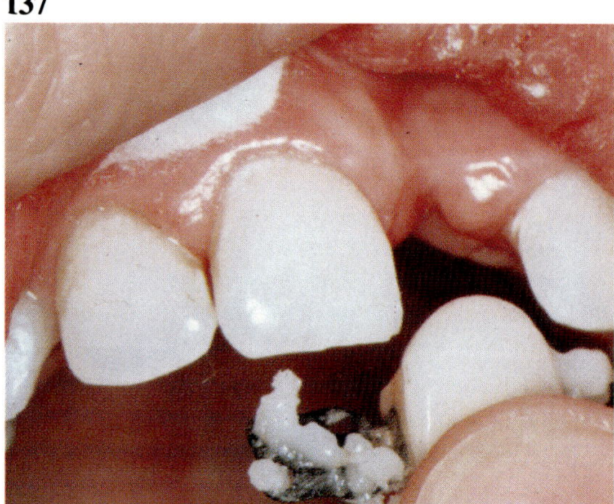

137 A chemically cured composite resin is then mixed and placed on the fitting surface of the bridge . . .

138

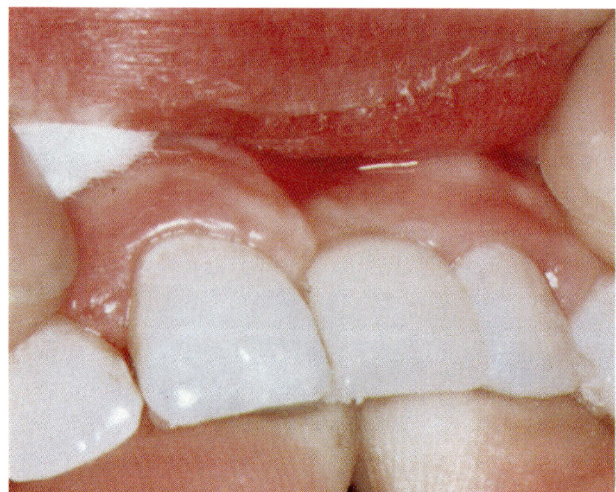

138 . . . which is then placed into position and held firmly for 5 minutes until polymerisation has been completed. It is essential that some composite flows through the holes and forms a thin film on the palatal surface of the bridge because this holds the bridge in position.

139

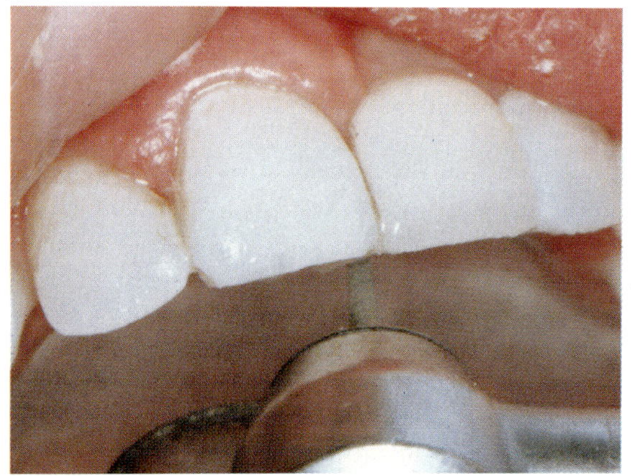

139 Any excess composite is trimmed away with a fine diamond bur.

140

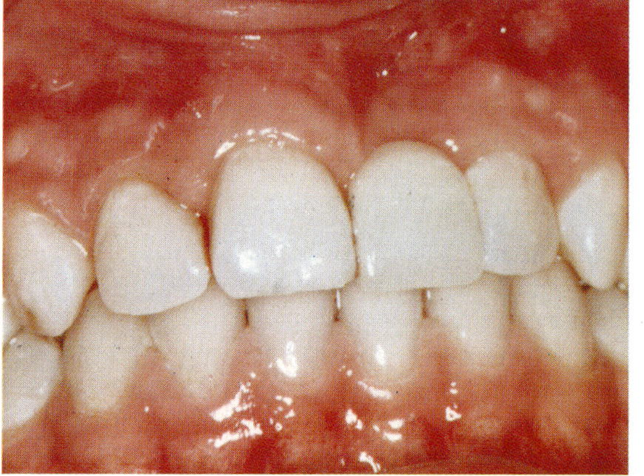

140 Labial view of the bridge in position

Note: The bridge framework is cast from precious or non-precious metal, and the pontic is built up from a compatible bonded porcelain. The composite bonds firmly to the tooth surface because of the millions of tags formed as a result of the acid etching and then holds the bridge in position by means of the film of composite squeezing through the holes in the wings onto the outer surface of the metal. A visible light curing composite is *unsuitable* because the light cannot shine through the metal and polymerise the composite on the fitting surface.

The acid etch retained bridge can be used to replace more than one tooth.

141

141 Patient with a denture replacing upper right central and lateral incisors.

142

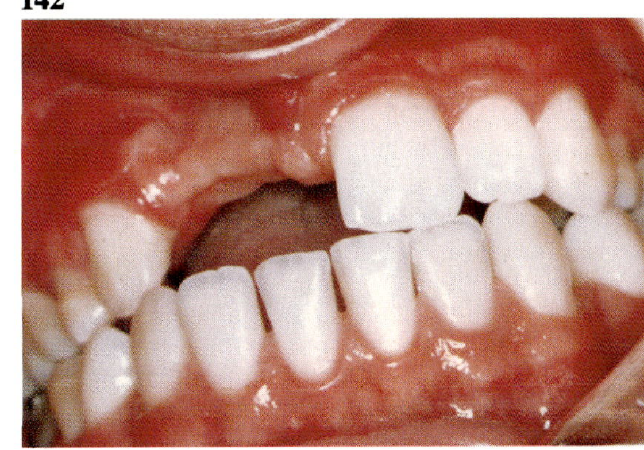

142 Labial view showing the missing teeth.

143

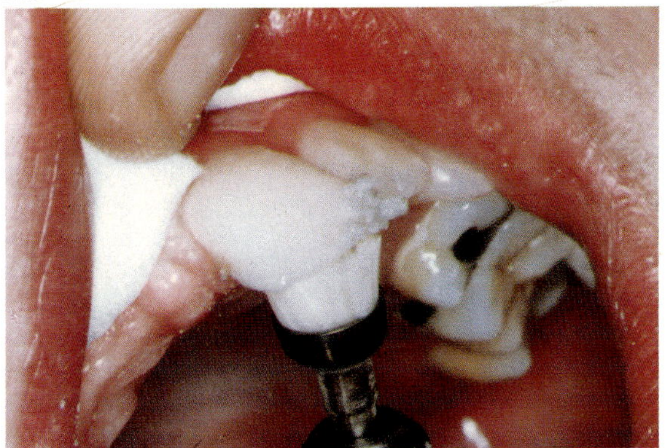

143 The palatal surfaces of the upper left central and lateral incisors and the upper right canine are cleaned . . .

144

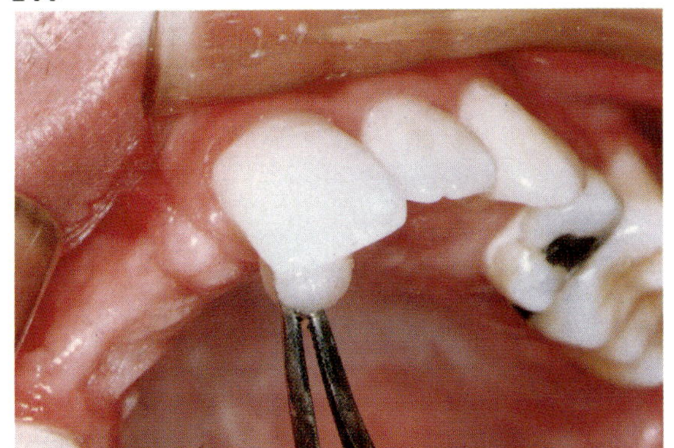

144 . . . etched, washed and dried . . .

145

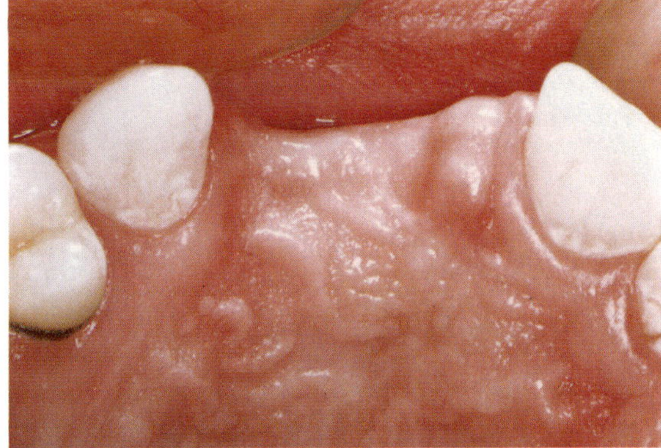

145 . . . to obtain a 'frosty' appearance on all three palatal surfaces.

A number of alternatives to making the 'wings' with holes to maintain the bridge in position have been proposed. In the 'Maryland System' the metal covering the abutment teeth is treated electrolytically to obtain a roughened finish on the fitting surface of the metal, similar to that obtained by acid etching the enamel surface. With the 'Duralingual System' a special wax mesh is placed on the working model which gives a mesh finish to the fitting surface of the metal work similar to that found on orthodontic attachments.

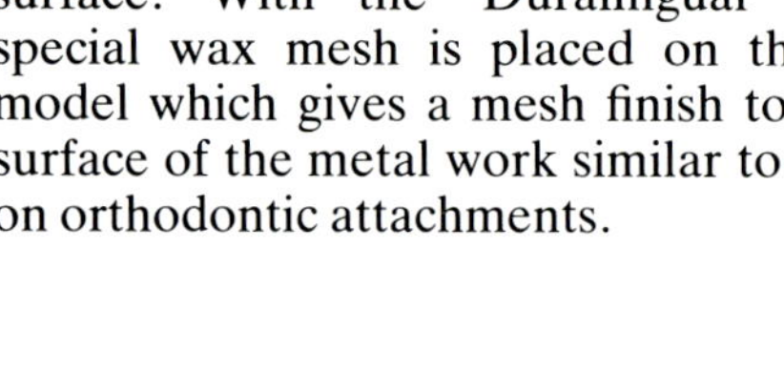

146

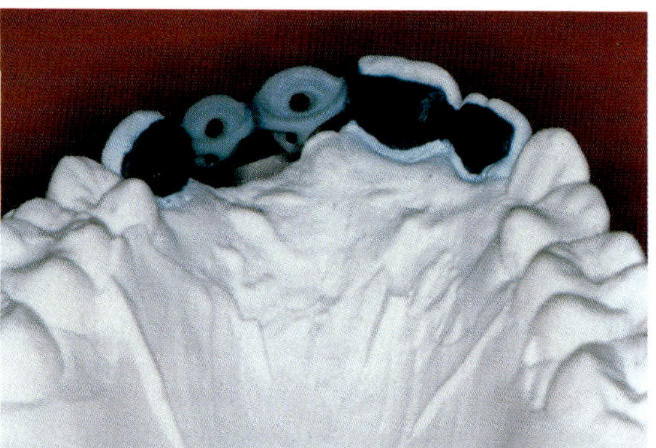

146 Wax pattern which is applied to the abutments, in the Duralingual system.

147

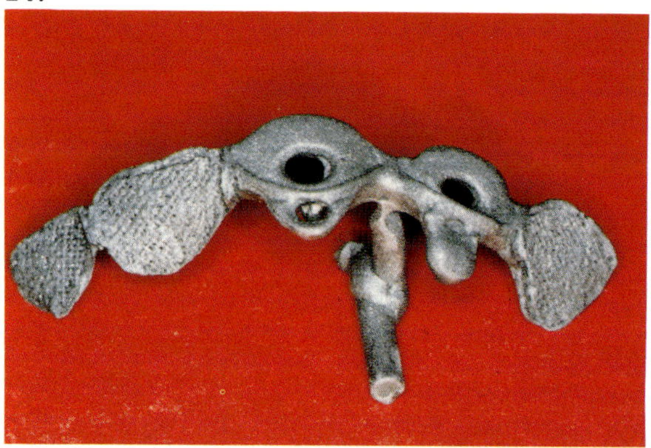

147 Fitting surface of the cast framework.

148

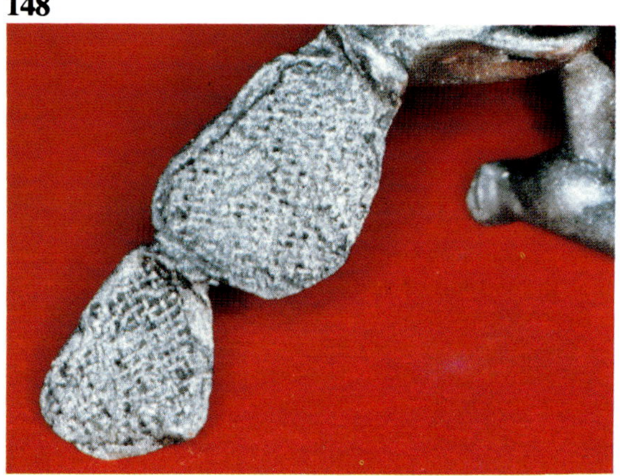

148 Close up of the fitting surface of one of the abutments.

149

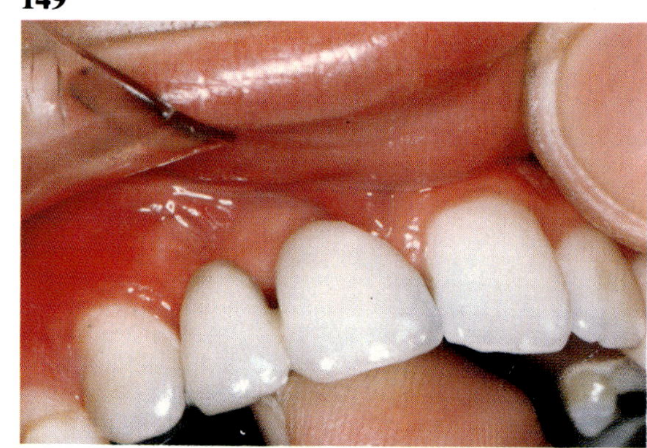

149 Labial view of bridge in position.

150

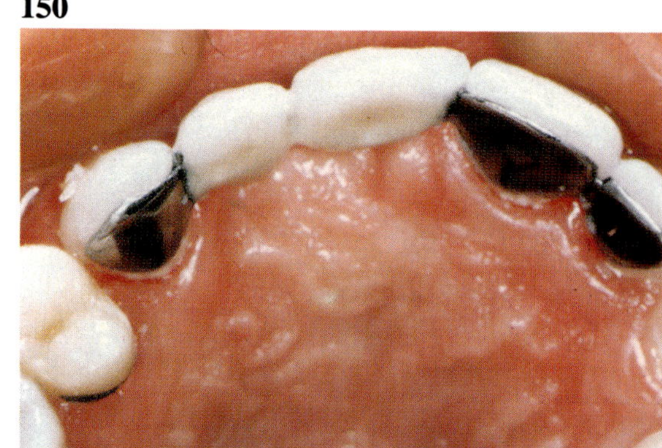

150 Palatal view of bridge showing the abutment on upper left central and lateral incisors and upper right canine.

151

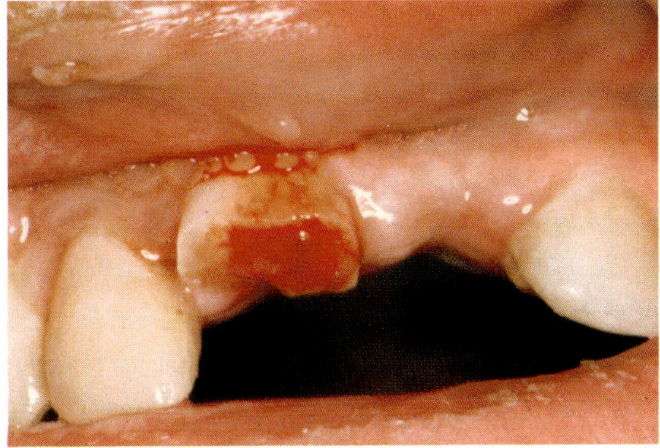

151 The general design can be varied. A patient who had a conventional 'Rochette Bridge' was hit in the face with a cricket bat, dislodging the bridge and fracturing the crown of the upper right central incisor.

152

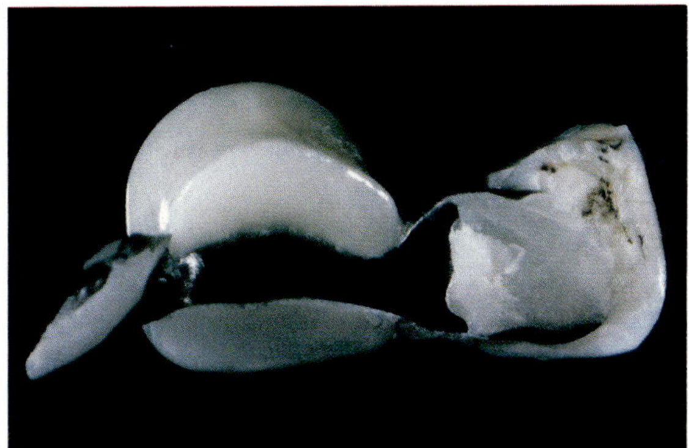

152 Palatal view of dislodged bridge, showing the 'butterfly' still adhering to the natural crown.

153

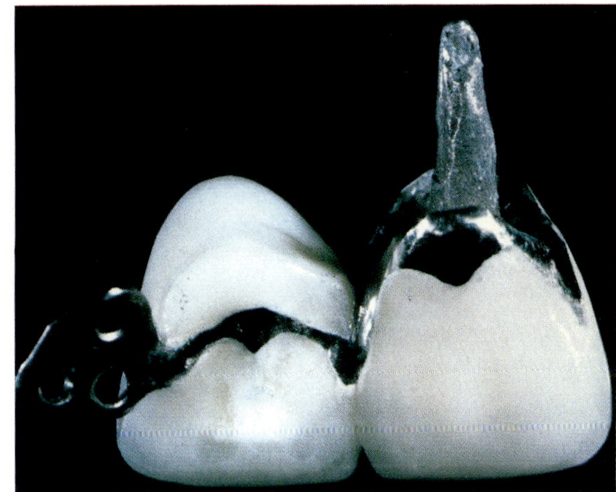

153 The upper right central incisor was root filled and a new bridge made incorporating a post crown on the root filled tooth.

154

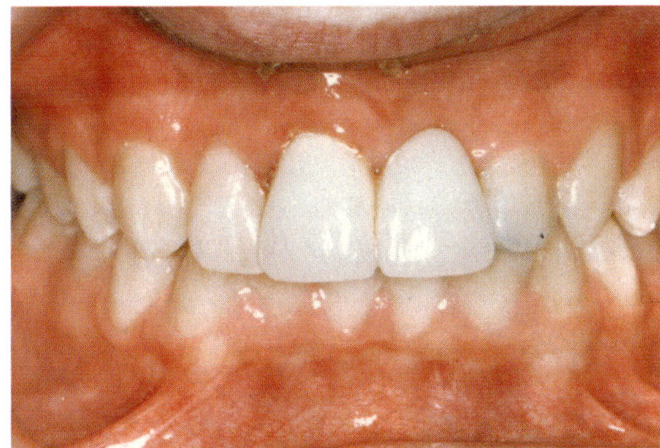

154 The bridge in position – labial view . . .

155

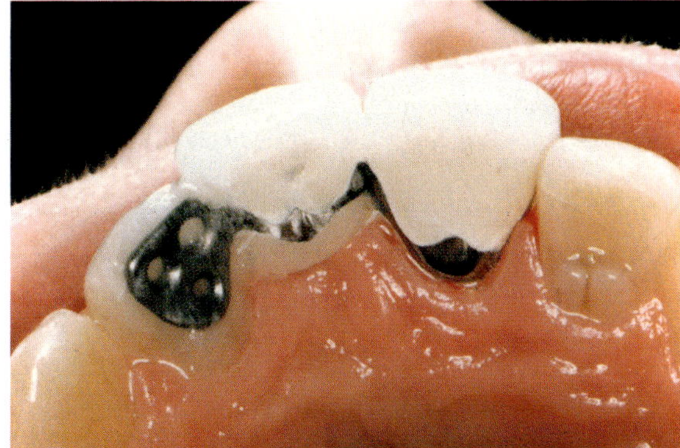

155 . . . and palatal view.

156

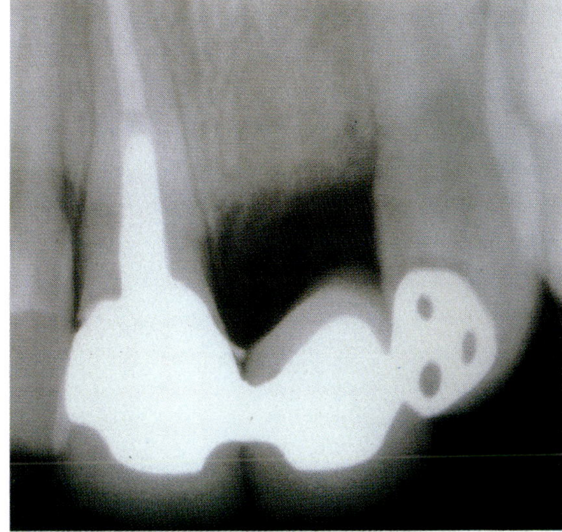

156 Radiograph of the bridge in position.

Malformed teeth

The developing crown of a permanent tooth can be damaged by trauma many years before it erupts. The emerging crown may be discoloured, or misshapen and can interfere with the occlusion.

157

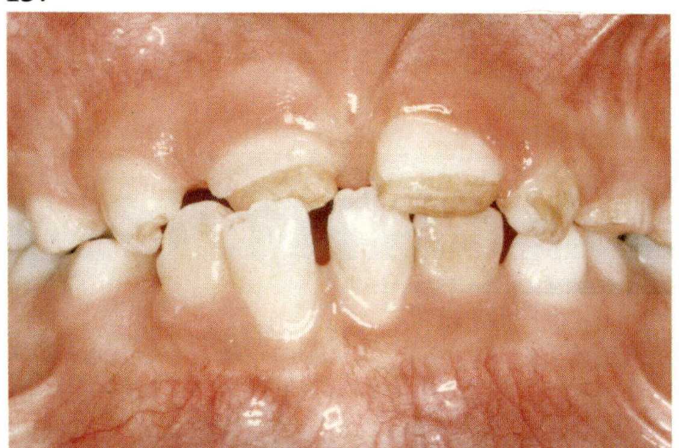

157 A child who had fallen when ten months old and loosened the upper deciduous incisors. The tips of the crowns of the upper permanent incisors were unsightly when they erupted at 8 years of age and the right central incisor is trapped behind the lower incisors.

158

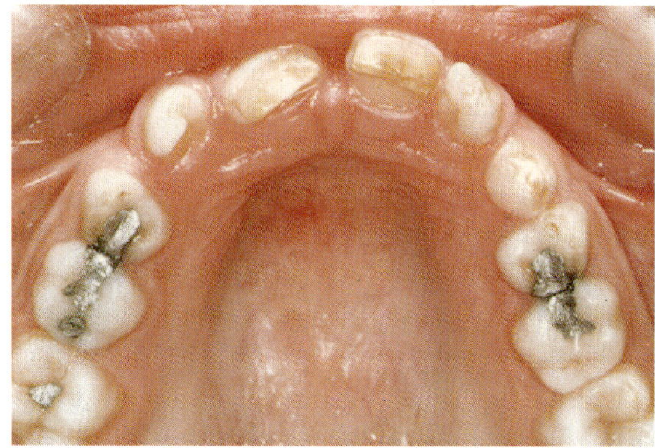

158 Palatal view, showing the affected incisal edges.

159

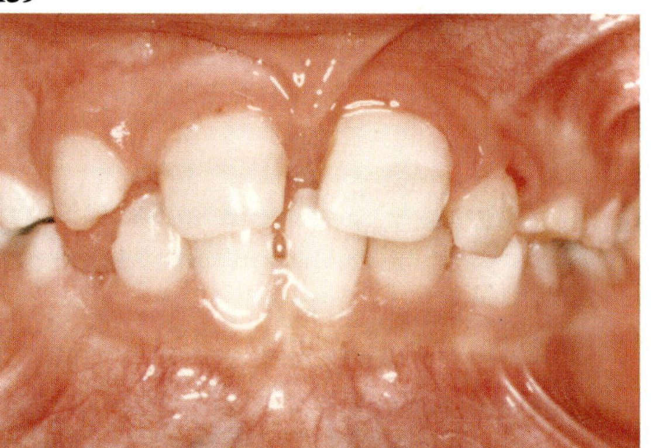

159 Labial view, showing composite restorations placed on all four upper incisors. The appearance and the occlusion have been improved.

160

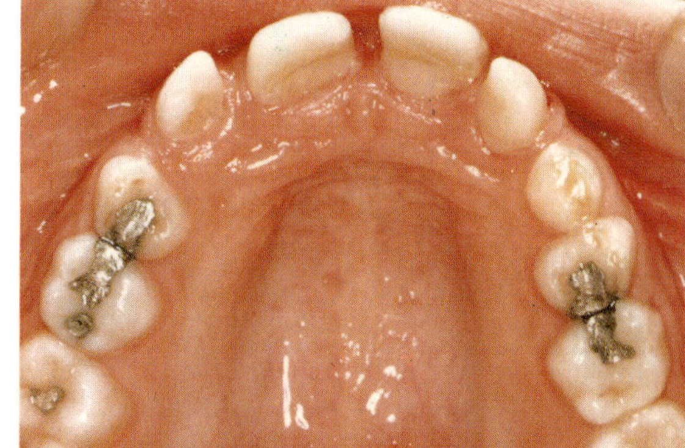

160 Palatal view of the case.

161

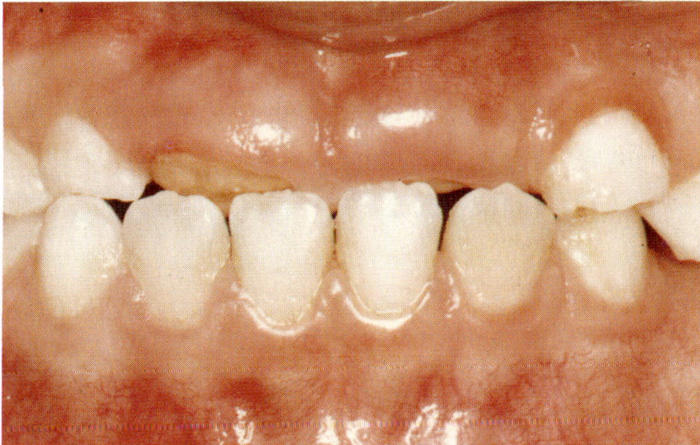

161 Labial view of a more severe case where the child fell at 18 months of age. The permanent incisors erupted when the child was almost 9 years old. The occlusion is such that permanent restorations would be impossible without orthodontic treatment and orthodontic treatment is extremely difficult because of the lack of a clinical crown.

162

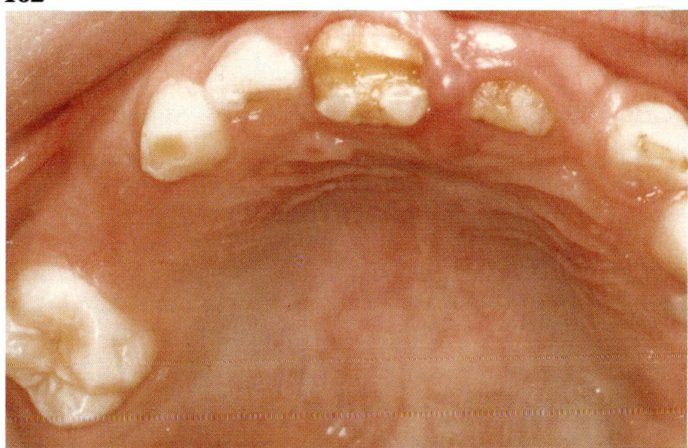

162 Palatal view showing the grossly distorted crown of the upper central incisors. The incisal edge of each tooth is 'bent back on itself' and is thick and bulbous. The lateral incisors are not so badly affected.

163

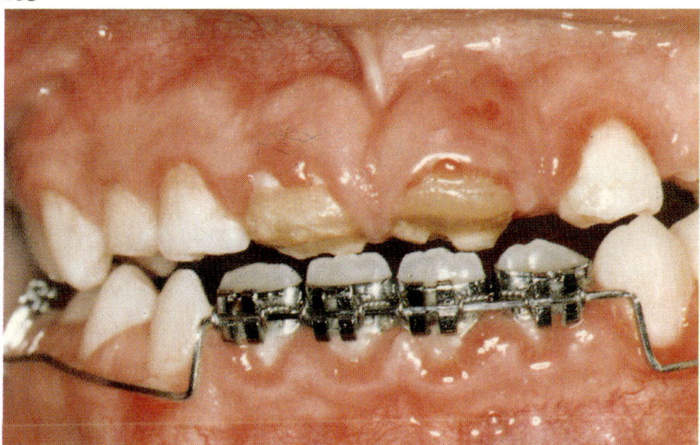

163 Orthodontic treatment carried out in the lower arch to depress the lower incisors and gain space for the provision of temporary crowns in the upper arch.

164

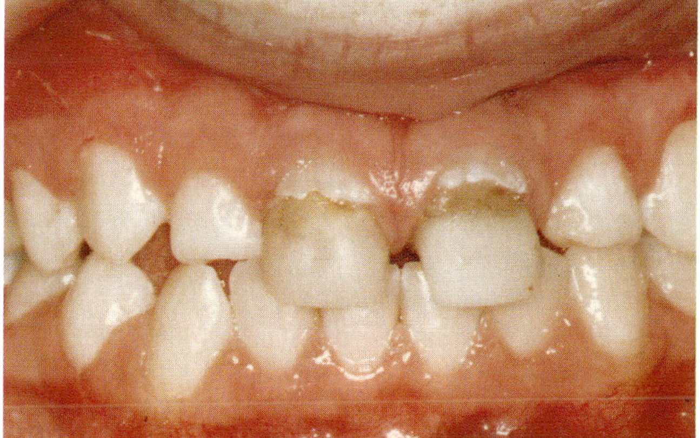

164 Temporary composite crowns bonded directly onto the available tooth substance (a mixture of enamel and dentine). These crowns have been in place for nearly 3 years.

165

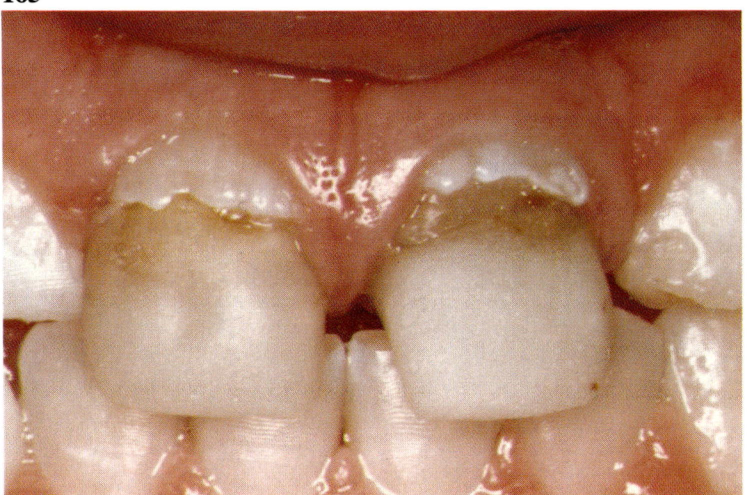

165 Close-up of temporary crowns. Although they are discoloured, particularly at the gingival margin, they did not become dislodged over the three year period.

166

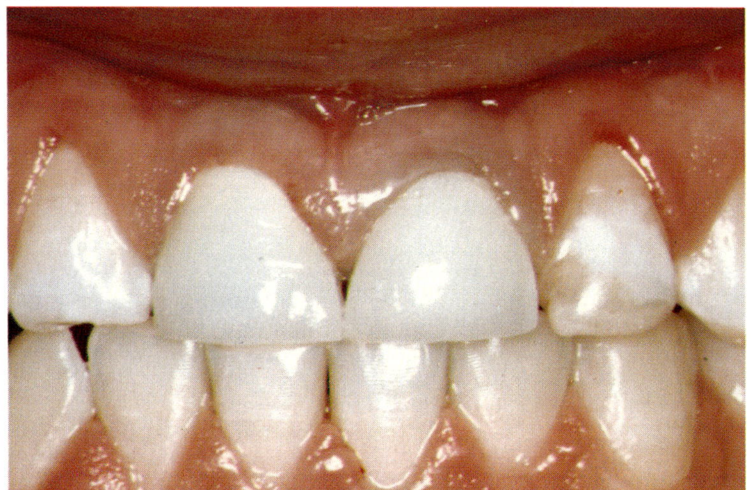

166 These teeth were root treated and post crowns made for the upper incisors – labial view . . .

167

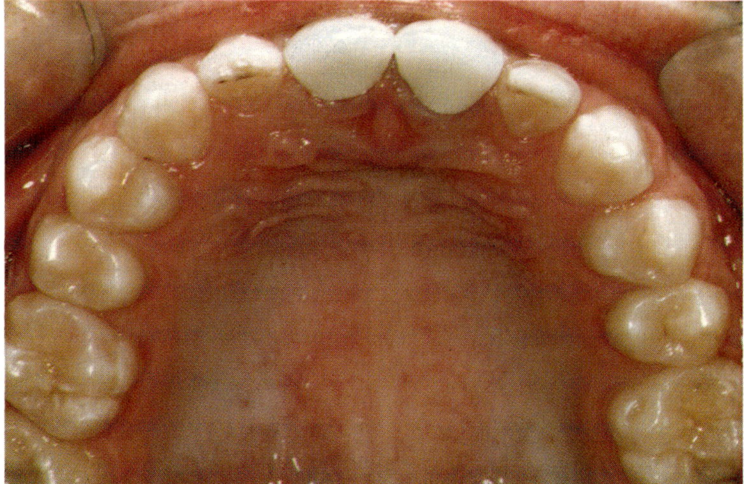

167 . . . and palatal view.

Direct bonding of orthodontic attachments

The bonding of orthodontic brackets directly onto the tooth surface has revolutionised the construction of fixed orthodontic appliances. Although the vital processes of diagnosis and treatment planning remain the prime factor in the success of any orthodontic treatment, the introduction of acid pre-treatment of the enamel surface, the development of composite adhesives, improvements in the design of brackets and the simplification of stock requirements, have all made life easier for both dentist and patient.

Fixed appliance therapy has been used for many years by specialist orthodontists for the treatment of severe malocclusions which are beyond the scope of this book. However, the use of bonded fixed appliances in less complicated cases enables the dentist to produce improvements in tooth position which could not easily be achieved with removable appliances. The cases to be described are all Class I malocclusions, where the aim was to improve the alignment of anterior teeth.

Although standard composites can be used for orthodontic purposes, manufacturers have also produced specially modified materials. In particular, the 'no-mix' materials are very convenient and their use will be described.

The direct bonding technique is not difficult to apply to anterior teeth but the various stages must be carried out precisely. It is more difficult to keep posterior teeth completely dry, and to position the attachments accurately, and therefore many orthodontists continue to use bands on molar teeth.

168

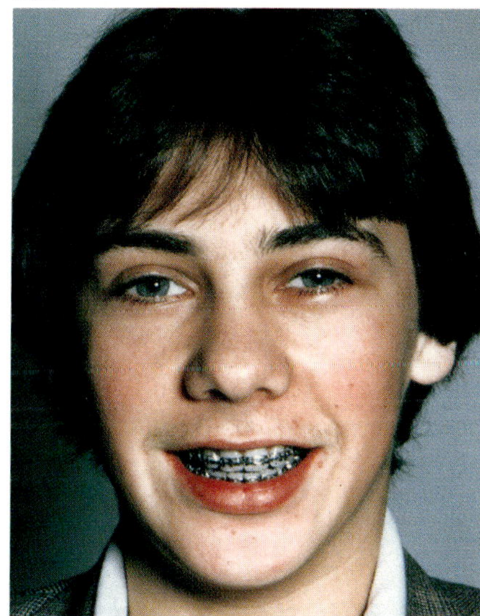

168 For a century or more, fixed appliances meant bands. In spite of the evolution of preformed bands with pre-welded attachments, banding was a considerable barrier to the use of fixed appliances by all except specialist orthodontists.

169

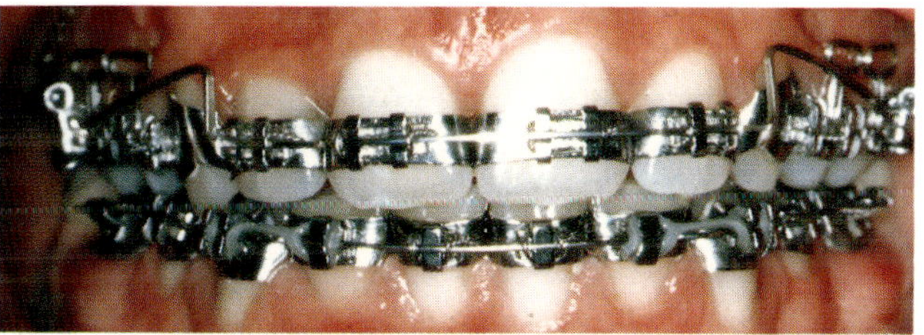

169 As the bands cover the full mesiodistal width of the teeth, relatively little enamel surface is visible and the overall effect is one of discoloration and greyness.

170

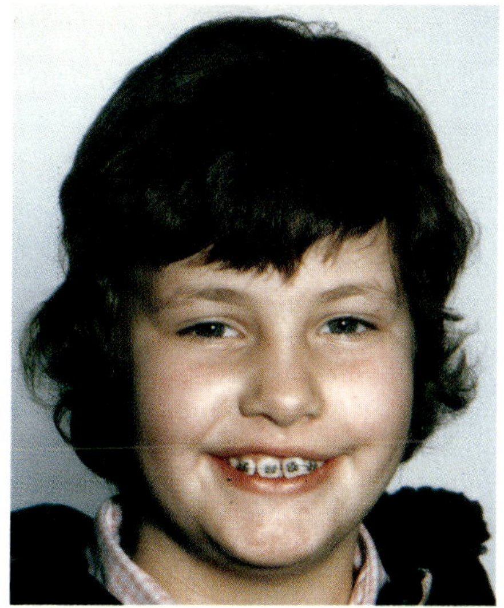

170 The main advantage in direct bonding, from the patient's point of view, is the improved appearance. The bracket is the same but the bonding pad covers a much smaller area of the enamel.

171

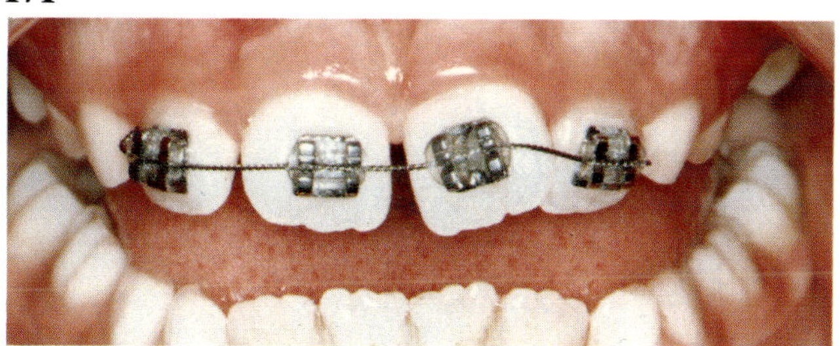

171 No part of the appliance passes between the teeth. Appointments to place the appliance are therefore more comfortable and shorter.

172

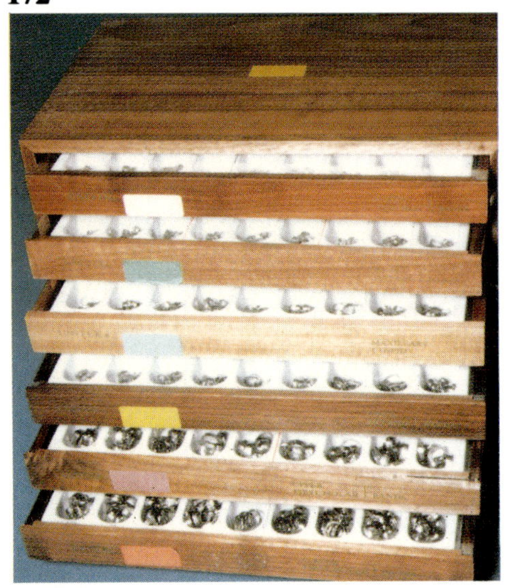

172 From the dentist's point of view there is no longer any need to stock large numbers of bands to fit every size and shape of tooth.

173

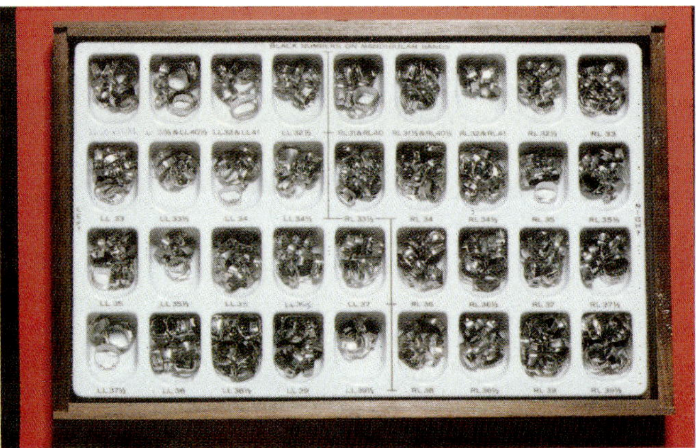

173 This box contains 42 different sizes of bands to fit upper left and upper right first permanent molars. Similar boxes were needed for all the other teeth. If each band carried a pre-welded attachment, a large capital outlay was involved.

174

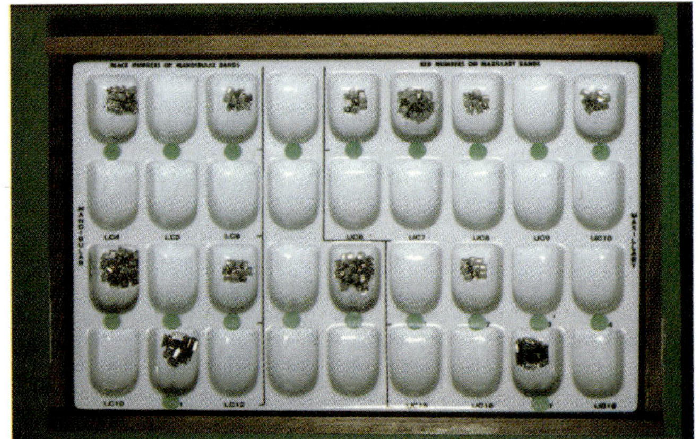

174 Brackets for bonding placed in a similar box, to show the relatively small stock which needs to be carried. Many bracket types are available. We suggest that three standard edgewise brackets with 0.45 mm (0.018″) slots should be stocked:

1 Medium width bracket on a flat base – upper central incisors.

2 Narrow bracket on a flat base – all other incisors.

3 Medium bracket on a curved base – canines and premolars.

175

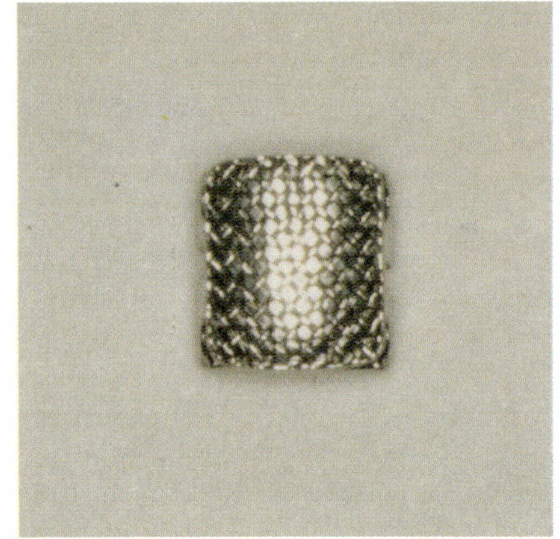

175 Close-up of fitting surface of bracket base to show one design of mesh for mechanical attachment of composite.

Direct bonding technique

The technique for the direct bonding of orthodontic brackets is similar to that already described for paedodontic procedures but with a few modifications.

Even though the oral hygiene is apparently satisfactory the teeth to be bonded should be polished to remove any residual plaque or staining. Pumice and water may be used or a proprietary oil-free, fluoride-free paste. Any blemishes on the tooth surfaces should be pointed out to patient and parent and recorded in the notes or photographed. The teeth should then be isolated either with cotton-wool rolls or special cheek retractors before etching the enamel surfaces. The etchant may be applied on a small pledget of cotton-wool or a mini-sponge. Thirty seconds is usually an adequate etching time, though manufacturers may suggest longer. At the end of the appropriate time it is essential that all the acid and breakdown products are removed by thorough washing with water for at least 20 seconds. The surfaces are then dried for 30 seconds.

After etching it is important that the enamel is kept isolated and that there is no saliva contamination. If this does occur, the tooth concerned should be thoroughly washed again, re-etched and dried. The enamel surface should now demonstrate the white 'frosty' appearance. If it does not, the etching procedure must be repeated. The etched area must be larger than the area of the bracket base so that all the adhesive is attached to etched enamel, otherwise there is a risk of decalcification underneath unbonded adhesive.

Adhesive resin is then applied with a brush to the back of the bracket and to the etched labial surface of the tooth. An appropriate quantity of the composite material is loaded onto the bracket base; the bracket is placed in position in the centre of the enamel surface, moved slightly from side to side to ensure an even layer of adhesive behind the bracket, then pressed firmly into position. A small excess of composite should be visible all round the bracket base. This excess should be smoothed to a feather edge against the tooth surface with a probe or similar instrument, before setting occurs. Over-zealous clearing of the excess may permit decalcification to occur immediately around the bracket even if the oral hygiene is apparently good. When all the brackets are in position, a few minutes should be allowed for the composite to harden before the arch wire is fitted.

Caution

All etching solutions contain acid, usually phosphoric acid. Avoid contact with eyes, skin, oral mucosa and dentine. In case of contact, wash immediately with water and seek medical attention if eyes are involved. Do not take internally.

Composite materials contain polymerisable monomers which may cause sensitisation or irritation if allowed to contact soft tissues. Wash thoroughly with soap and water if contact occurs. Do not use if there is a known allergy to methacrylate resin.

176

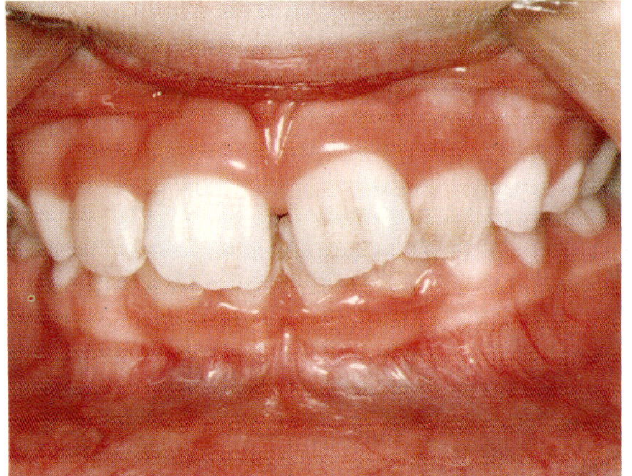

176 The tilt and rotation of /1 make a simple fixed appliance appropriate.

177

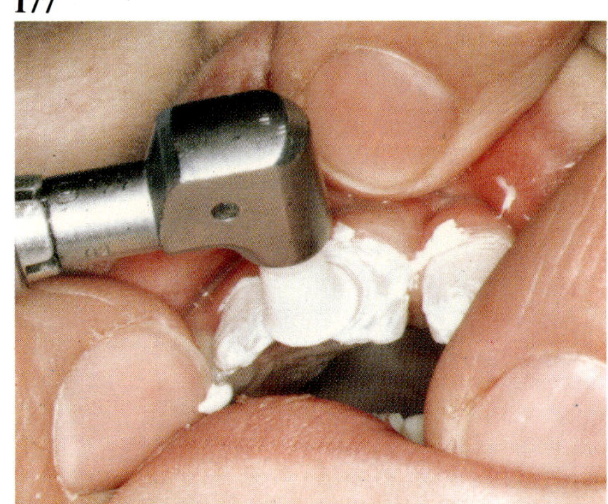

177 Polish with oil-free, fluoride-free paste to remove any plaque or stain.

178

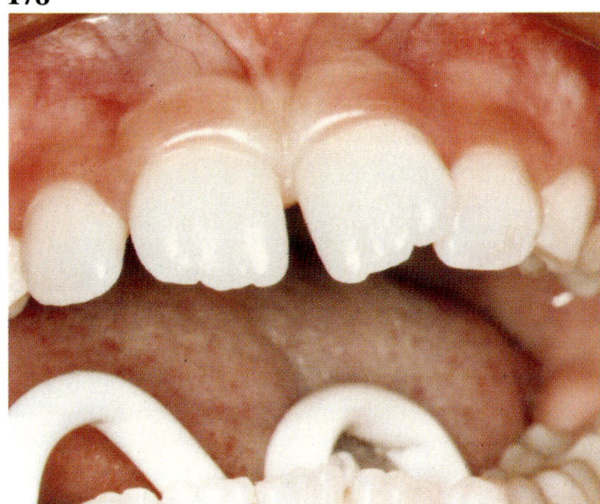

178 Teeth cleaned and isolated, ready for etching.

179

179 Apply etchant, with small cottonwool pledget or mini-sponge, for 30 to 60 seconds.

180

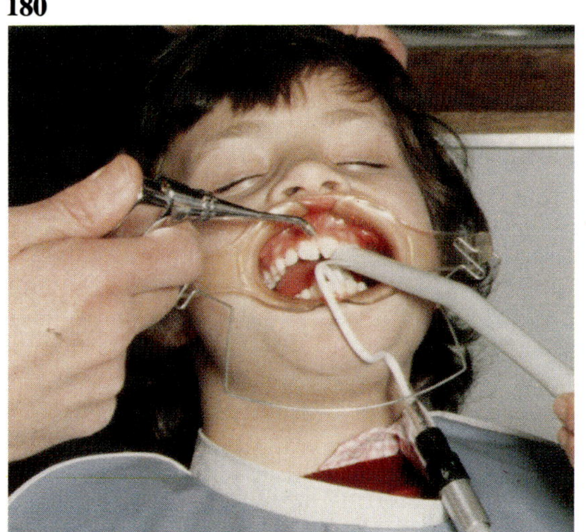

180 Wash all the etched surfaces quickly to stop most of the acid activity. Then wash thoroughly for at least 20 seconds to remove all trace of etchant and breakdown products.

181

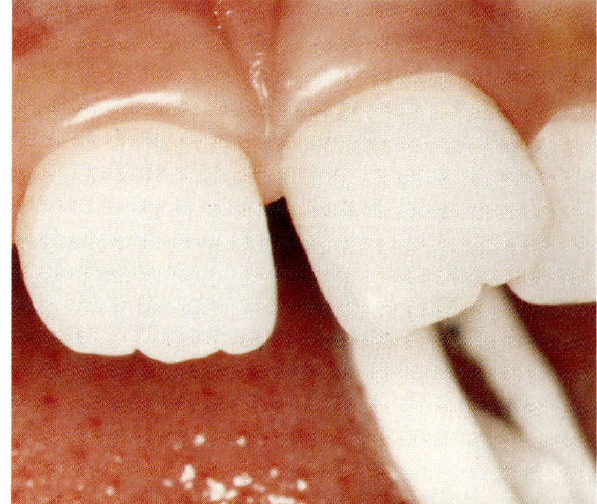

181 Enamel surfaces dried for 30 seconds and ready for bonding. Note the 'frosty' appearance.

182

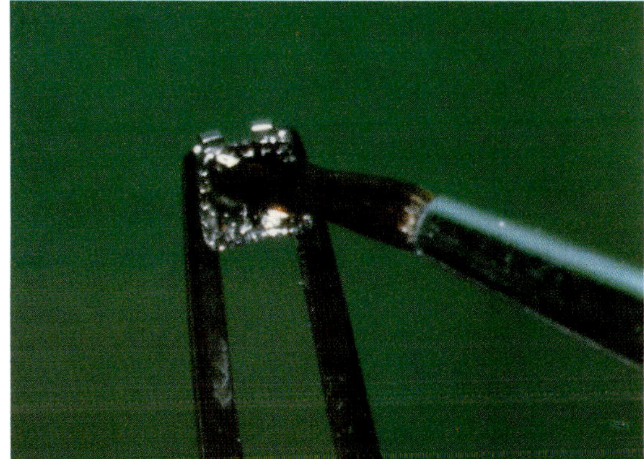

182 Apply resin to the bracket base.

183

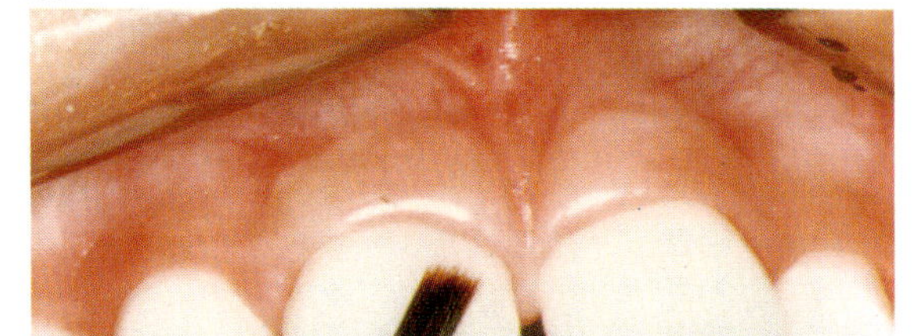

183 Apply resin to the prepared enamel surface.

184

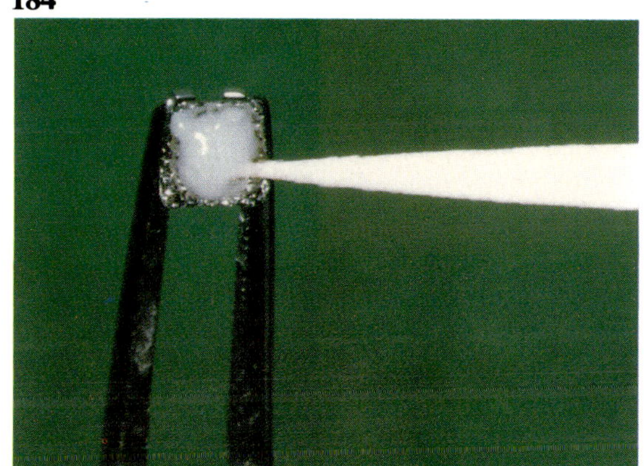

184 Apply bonding composite material to bracket base.

185

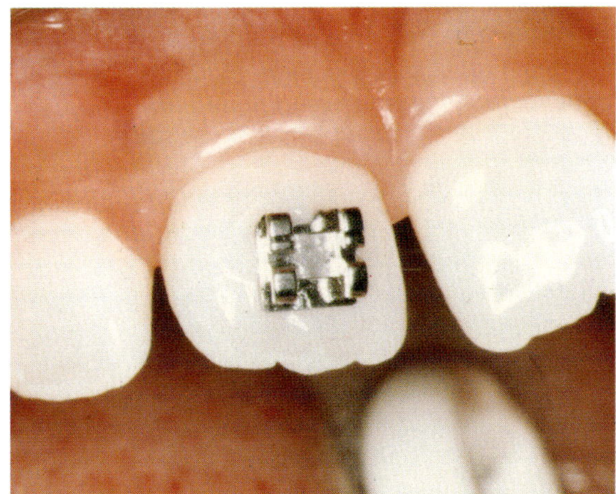

185 Place bracket in centre of labial surface and slide gently into correct position. Press bracket firmly against the tooth. A small excess of material should be present.

186

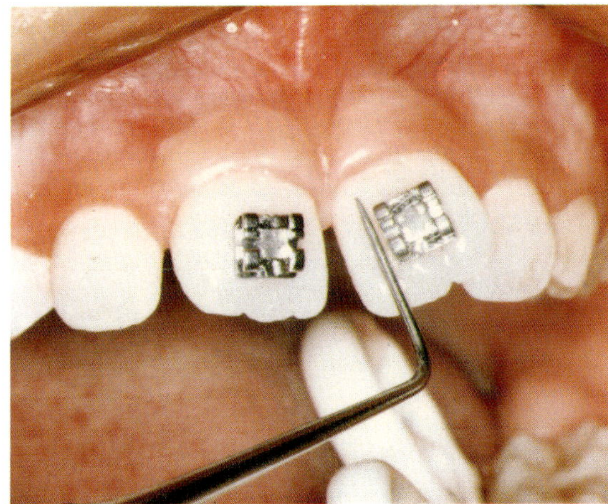

186 Probe demonstrates relationship of bracket to long axis of tooth. The excess bonding material is smoothed to a feather edge.

187

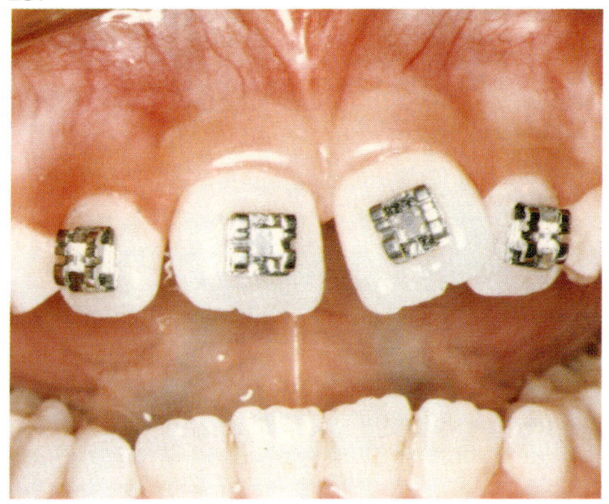

187 Brackets in position on 21/12. If, in spite of careful technique, a bracket comes loose during treatment, any residual adhesive should be removed from the enamel before the bonding procedure is repeated.

Rotation and alignment of anterior teeth

(a) Sectional fixed appliance

It is often possible to rotate and align anterior teeth using only a small number of brackets. These must be bonded to the teeth to be moved and to at least one correctly aligned tooth on each side of them.

The first wire, which can be placed within a few minutes of bonding, must be very flexible and a multistrand wire is often used. It should be formed into a curve to represent the arch shape and this curve may be slightly exaggerated to overcome the tendency for the teeth at the ends of the wire to flare labially. The ends of the wire should extend for 2 to 3mm beyond the last brackets and should be bent gingivally, before the wire is inserted, to avoid traumatising the lip. The wire is attached to the brackets by means of plastic modules which engage in the undercuts under the wings of the brackets. Before allowing the patient to leave the surgery instruction must be given in the care of the appliance.

Appointments are arranged at approximately monthly intervals and at each one the wire should be removed, the brackets checked for firmness and the oral hygiene also checked. Any areas of plaque accumulation should be pointed out to the patient. A fresh multistrand arch may be placed in a similar way, or if sufficient movement has occurred it may be possible to progress to a solid wire 0.35mm (0.014 inches) in diameter which should also be curved to the arch shape. Wherever possible, it is desirable to bend the wire to produce some overcorrection of rotations, as these are much more likely to relapse than other movements.

188

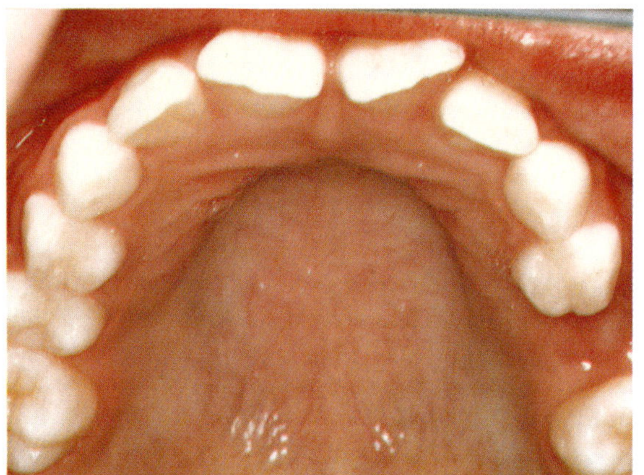

188 Occlusal view shows rotation of upper anterior teeth (same case as 176 to 187).

189

189 Multistrand wire in position at the end of the first visit. The clear plastic modules holding the wire into the brackets are just visible.

190

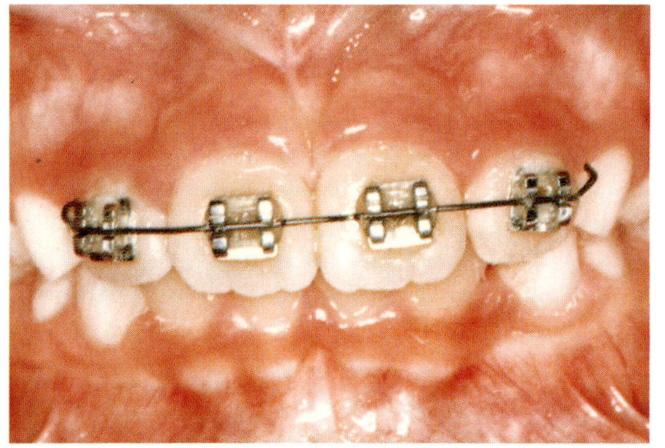

190 0.35 mm (0.014″) wire three months later.

191

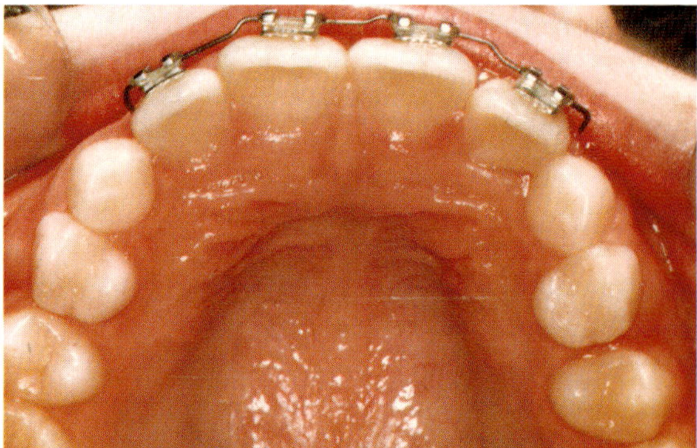

191 Occlusal view shows detail of wire bends. There are small lateral incisor insets and another bend between 1/1 to move /1 slightly labial to 1/ to over-correct the rotation.

192

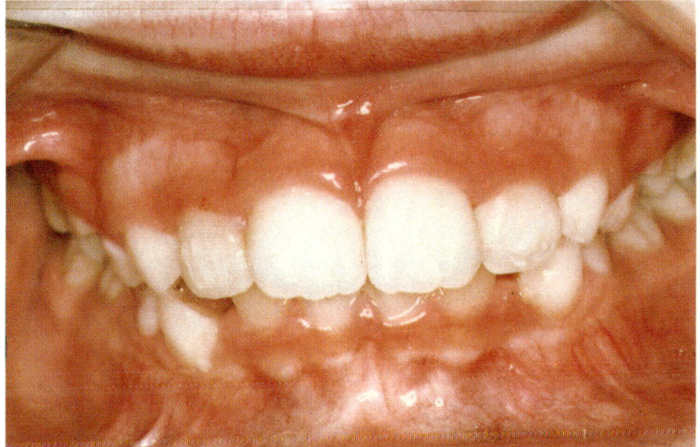

192 Immediately after removal of the fixed appliance. Traces of adhesive are still visible.

193

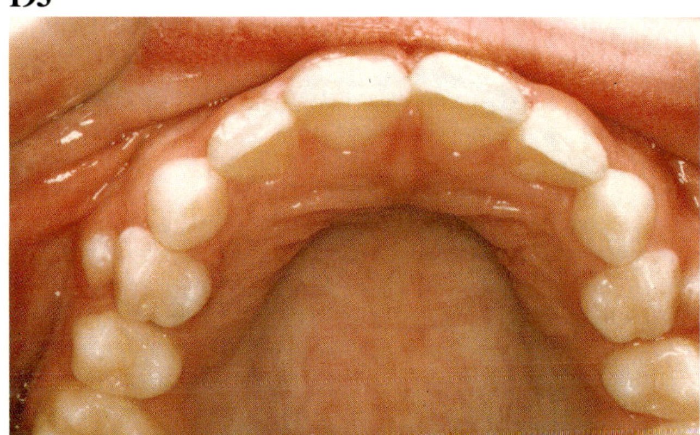

193 Occlusal view shows some over-correction of $\underline{/1}$.

194

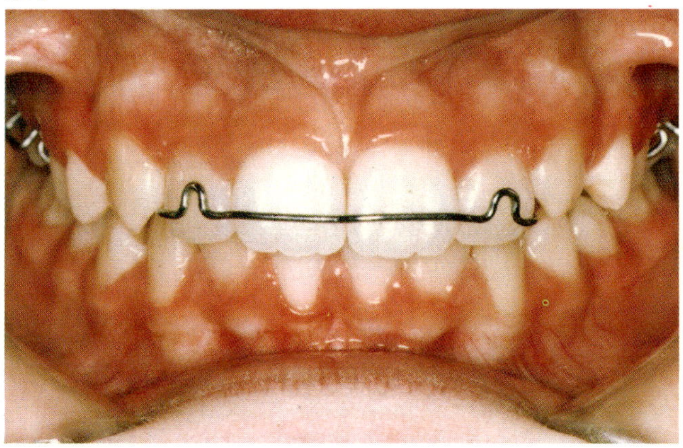

194 Removable appliance used as retainer.

195

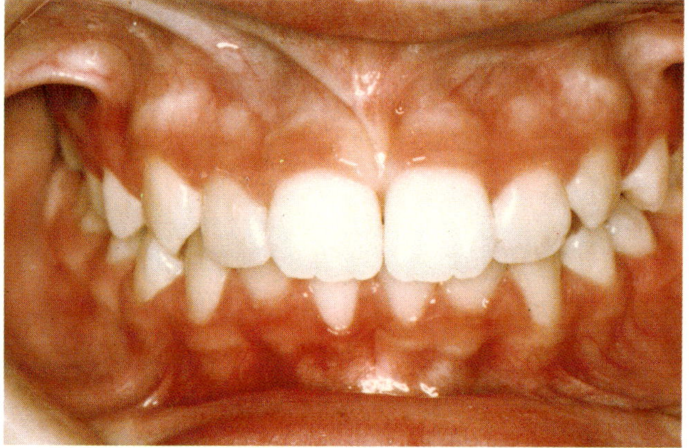

195 Six months after removal of the fixed appliance, the enamel surfaces look perfectly normal.

(b) The whip spring

196 Whip spring. This spring is used in conjunction with a removable appliance to treat a severely rotated tooth.

In this case, a bracket is bonded to the centre of the labial surface of the rotated central incisor. A short length of wire, with a hook at the end, is attached to the bracket and the hook is latched onto a wire component on the removable appliance thus creating a rotational force.

In spite of its apparent simplicity, there are many points to consider in the bending of a whip spring.

1 **Attachment to the bracket.** The wire does not pass through the bracket slot but fits under the four wings which are usually used for the plastic module. In the example shown, the wire passes under the gingival wings, down the mesial side of the bracket and back under the occlusal wings where a small loop is formed. A ligature is then applied across the distal side of the bracket to hold the whip spring in position.

2 **The wire itself** is 0.4 mm (0.016″) round wire spanning two teeth between the bracket and the hook.

3 **The hook** must be bent so that the whip stays in position except when the patient unlatches it. In this example, the rotation and distal tilt of the central incisor necessitate the hook being bent downwards and inwards. Care must be taken to prevent the end of the wire irritating the cheek: it should be short and on the gingival side of the hook.

4 **The free span of wire** must not contact any tooth between the bracket and the hook. If it does, the rotated tooth will be displaced labially.

5 **When a tooth is severely rotated** it is all too easy to apply an excessive force, causing discomfort and possible damage to the root of the tooth. Activation should be reduced by contouring the wire so that the hook is only 6 to 8 mm from the removable appliance wire.

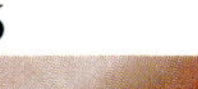
196

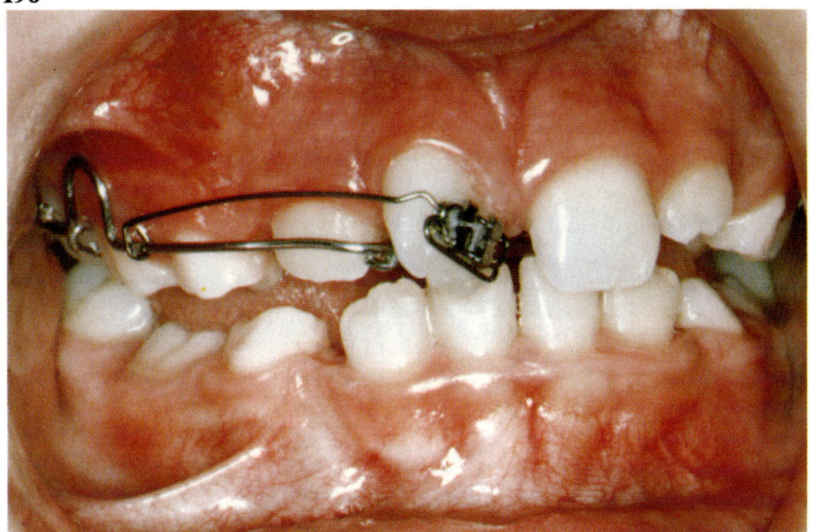

197

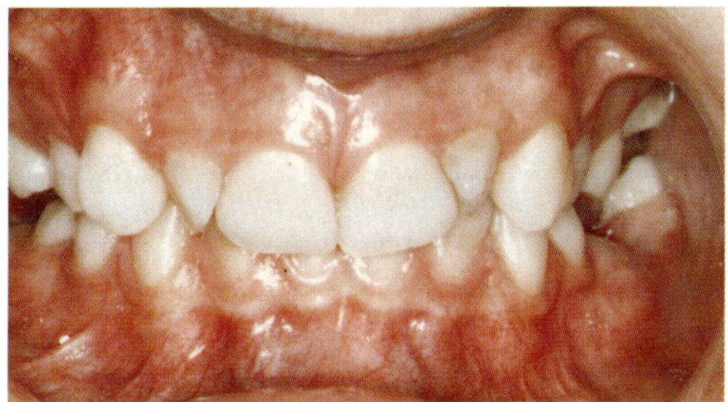

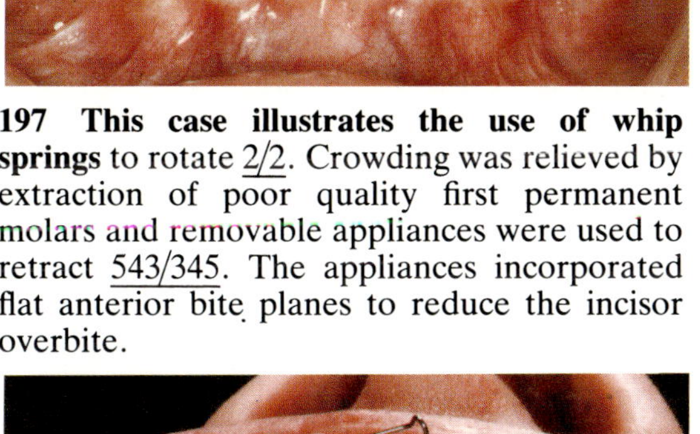

197 This case illustrates the use of whip springs to rotate 2/2. Crowding was relieved by extraction of poor quality first permanent molars and removable appliances were used to retract 543/345. The appliances incorporated flat anterior bite planes to reduce the incisor overbite.

198

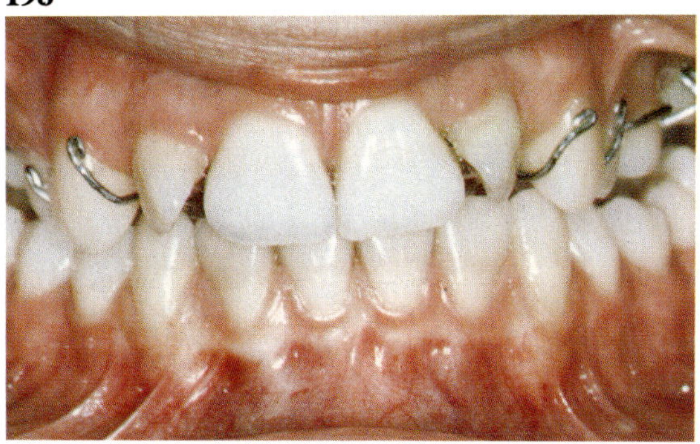

198 After retraction of 3/3.

199

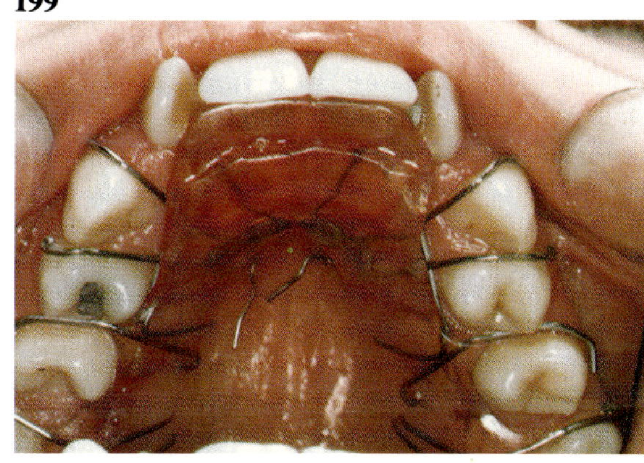

199 Space available for rotation of 2/2.

200

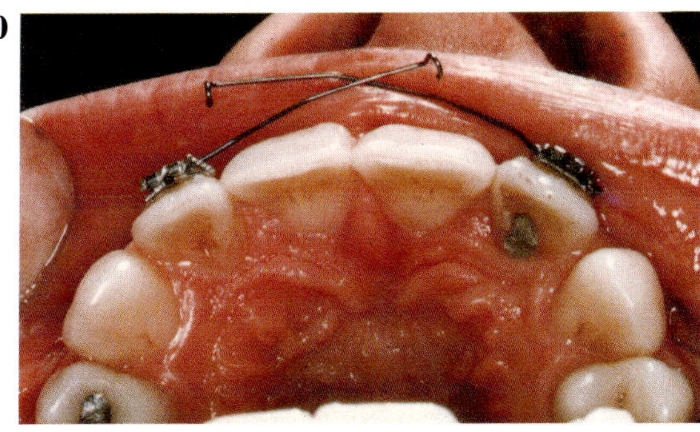

200 Occlusal view after rotation of 2/2 shows brackets bonded to 2/2 and whip springs in position, without the removable appliance.

201

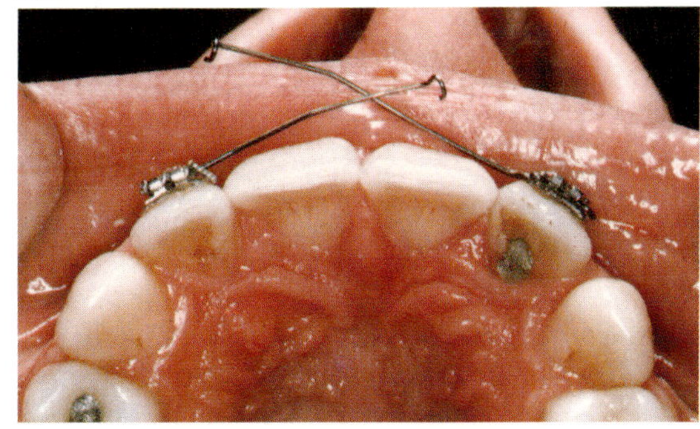

201 Incorrect bending of /2 whip. Contact between the wire and /1 would displace /2 labially.

202

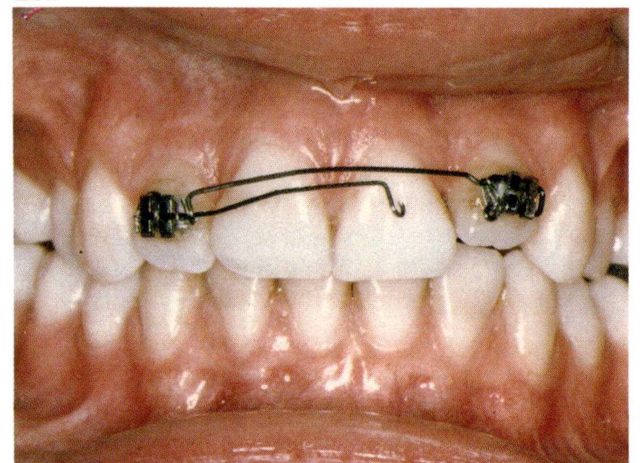

202 Anterior view without removable appliance.

203

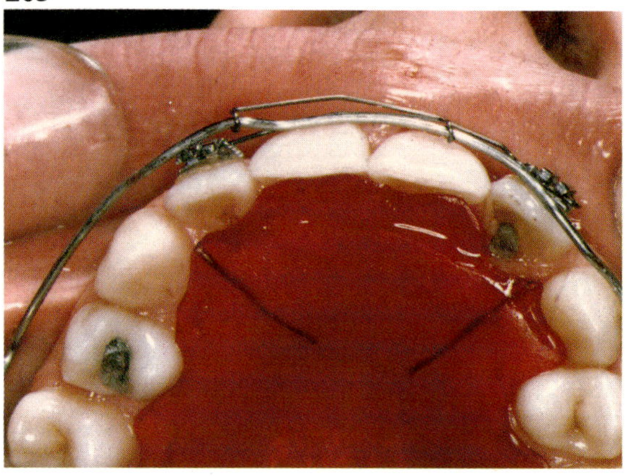

203 Hooks engaged onto labial bow. Each hook must be free to move along the wire as its tooth rotates.

204

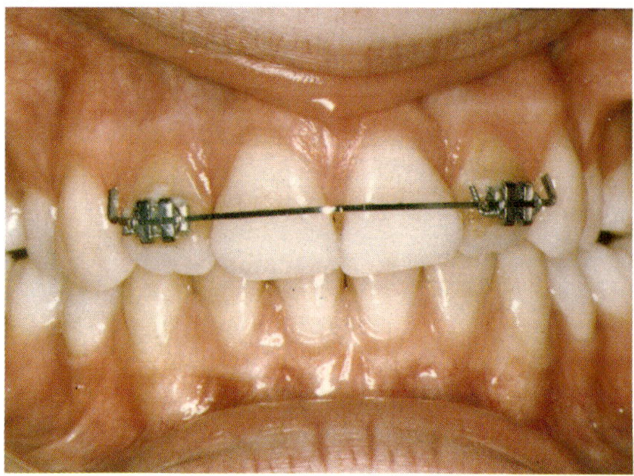

204 The initial period of retention can be carried out by joining the two brackets with a heavier archwire.

205

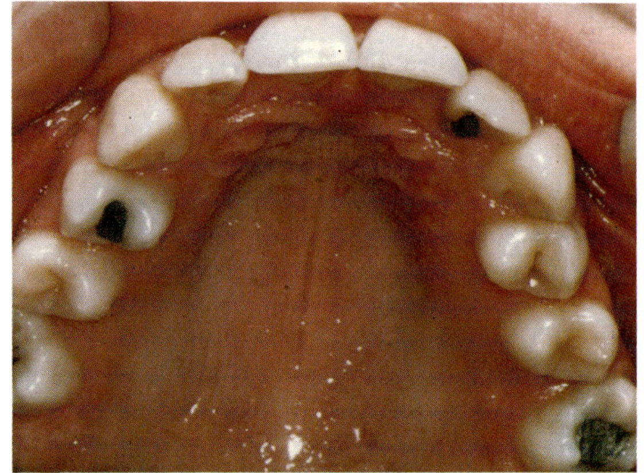

205 Occlusal view of result. Some over-rotation of the lateral incisors is visible.

206

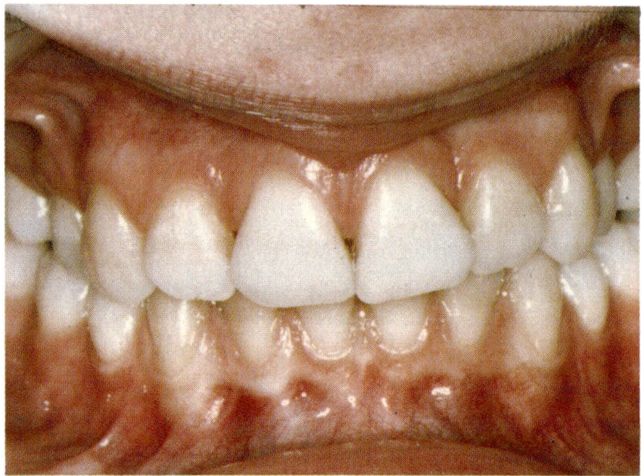

206 Anterior view of result. Retention must be continued for at least one year. In this case a removable appliance was used.

Treatment of ectopic incisors

An upper permanent incisor may be severely displaced, usually because of the presence of a supernumerary tooth. This should be recognised at an early stage, when the incisors are erupting; if one central incisor fails to erupt within a few months of the contralateral tooth, or if the lateral incisor erupts before the central, a radiograph should be taken of the unerupted tooth. Any supernumerary tooth should be removed, following which there may be natural eruption of the displaced incisor.

Unfortunately, some patients do not present for treatment until the age of 11 or 12 years when there is little alternative but to carry out surgical exposure and orthodontic alignment. It is not possible to carry out this tooth movement with a removable appliance on its own, but traction can be applied to the tooth by means of a vertical elastic from a bonded attachment on the labial surface of the affected tooth running to a wire on a removable appliance. The force applied must be small, perhaps 25 grams, and a latex elastic extended by 50 per cent would be suitable. As the tooth moves downwards smaller elastics are needed.

207

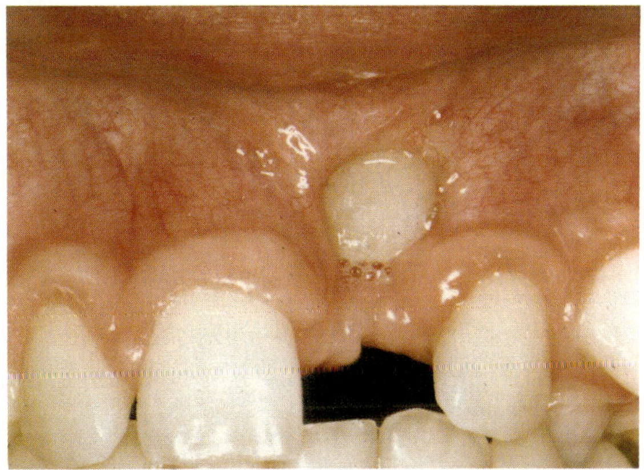

207 Soon after removal of the supernumerary teeth and surgical exposure of the upper left central incisor in a patient aged twelve years.

208

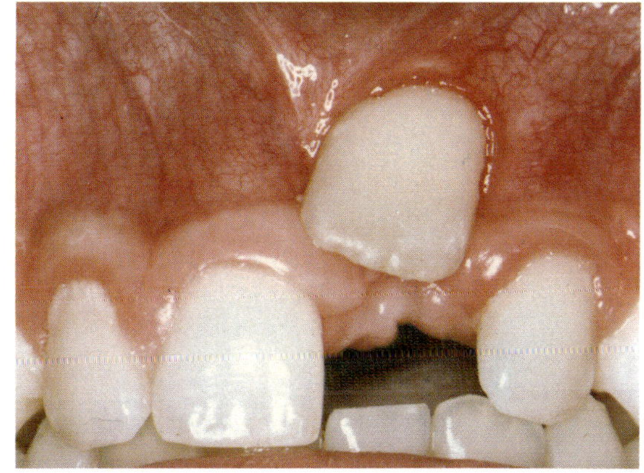

208 Almost one year later there has been very little further eruption.

209

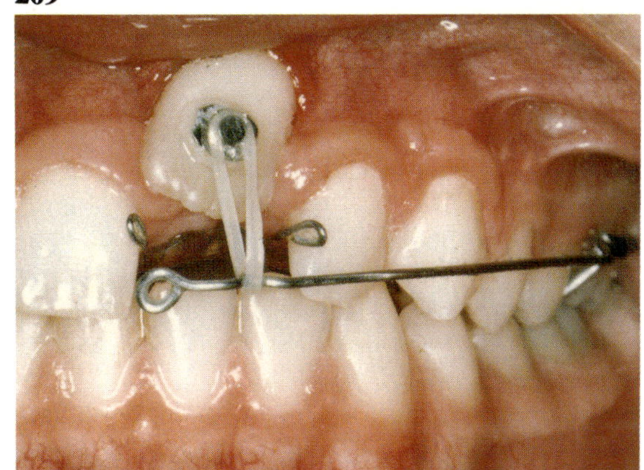

209 Attachment bonded into position with a vertical latex elastic running to a removable appliance. A shallow button has been used instead of a bracket, to minimise irritation to the inner surface of the lip. (Springs to open the space for the ectopic incisor are also visible.)

210

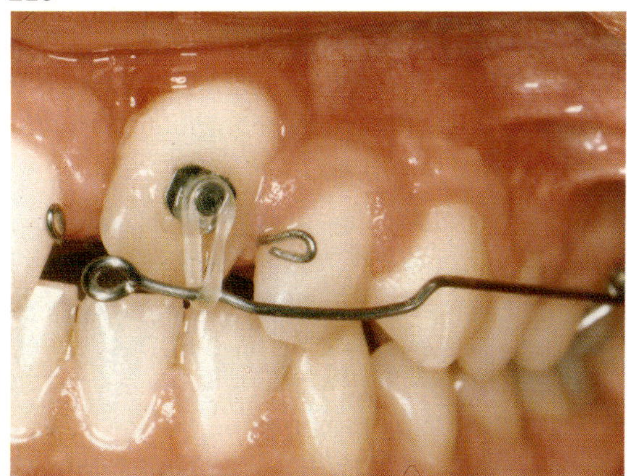

210 Four months later the tooth is approaching the occlusal level but some rotation is evident.

211

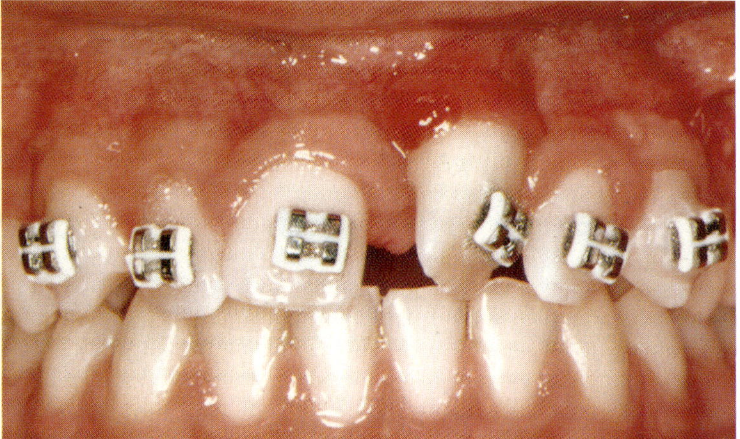

211 Brackets placed, before alignment. To prevent excess composite flowing into the bracket channels white bracket guards have been used. They are removed as soon as the composite has set.

212

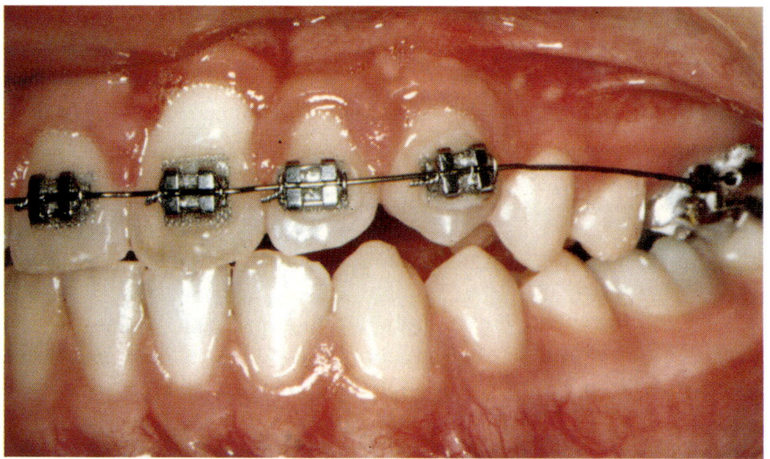

212 The upper canines flared buccally during this treatment. To correct this bands were placed on the upper first molars and a full upper archwire was used.

213

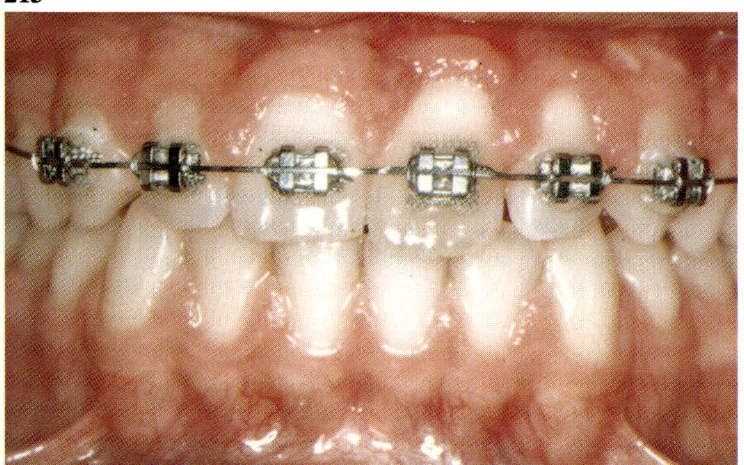

213 At the end of active treatment. Note that the incisal edge of the left central incisor is over-corrected to a position slightly below the other teeth.

214

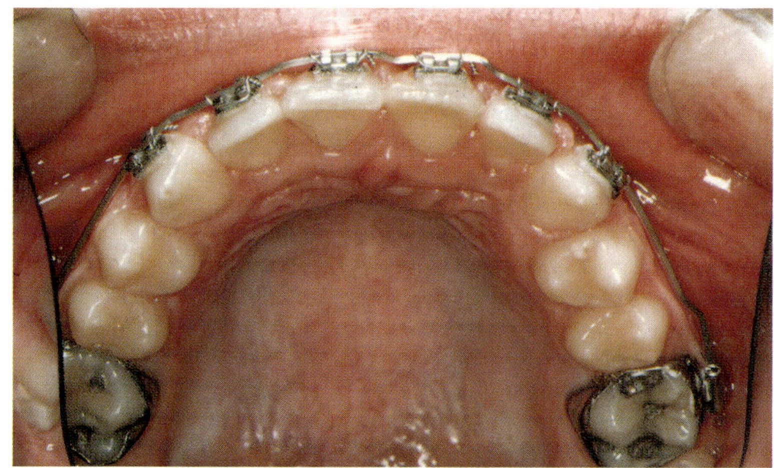

214 Occlusal view shows details of the bends in the archwire to correct the rotation of the left central incisor.

215 Anterior view after removal of brackets. The difference in gingival level of the upper incisors is a complication of the surgical exposure.

215

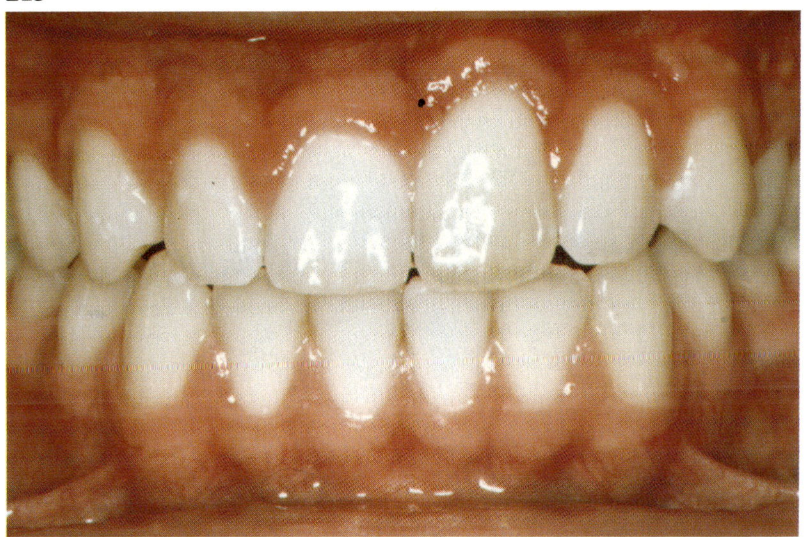

216 Occlusal view shows good alignment.

216

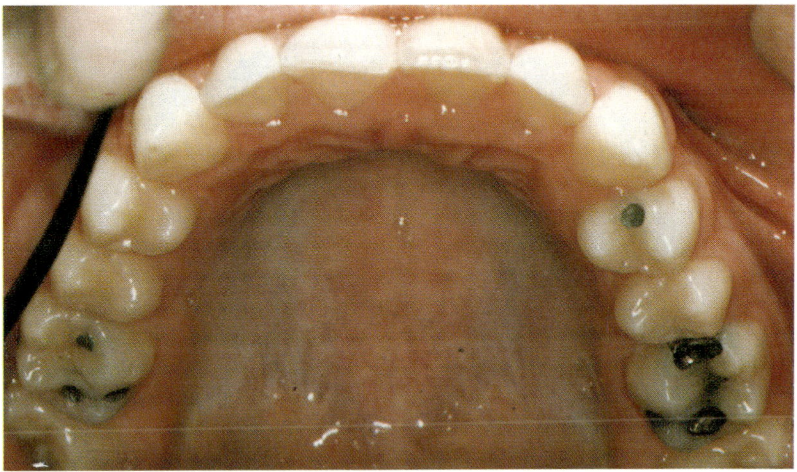

Treatment of palatal canines

Palatal displacement of the upper permanent canine tooth occurs in 1.5 to 2 per cent of the population. Suspicion of this should be aroused clinically if the tooth is not palpable in the buccal sulcus at age 9 or 10 years. If the tooth has not erupted at the same time as the contralateral tooth, or within a few months of the eruption of the first premolars, radiographs should be taken to confirm the presence and position of the unerupted canine. In the first instance, parallax views are helpful but if the tooth is shown to be palatal then further views will be needed to localise its position exactly.

Where the tooth is not excessively displaced, surgical exposure followed by orthodontic alignment is the treatment of choice for a good long-term prognosis. After surgical exposure the tooth may erupt spontaneously but usually an appliance is needed to move it buccally into the line of the arch. A bond may be placed on the accessible surface of the exposed tooth and an elastic used with a removable appliance in a similar way to that described for the ectopic incisor. Once the tooth is in the line of the arch further treatment may be needed to achieve full alignment.

217

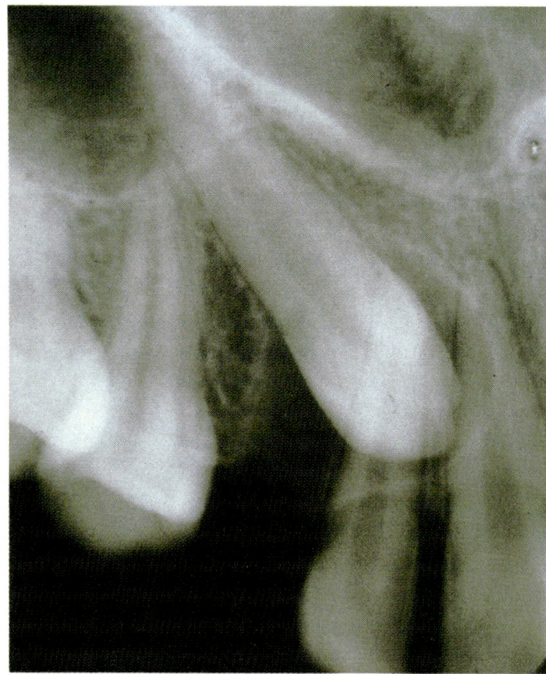

218

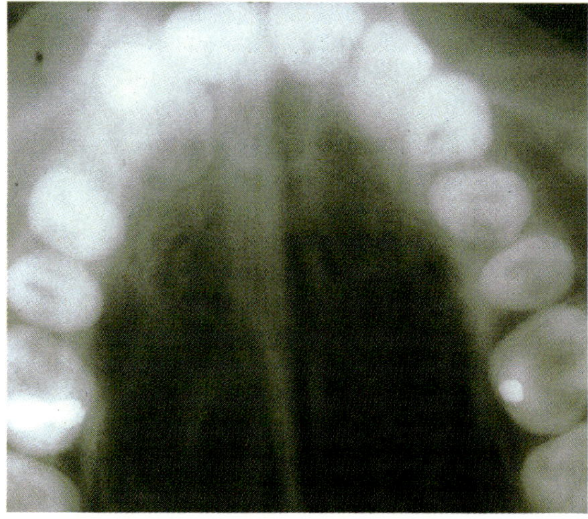

217 Intraoral xray shows the displaced upper right canine.

218 Vertex occlusal radiograph confirms palatal displacement.

219

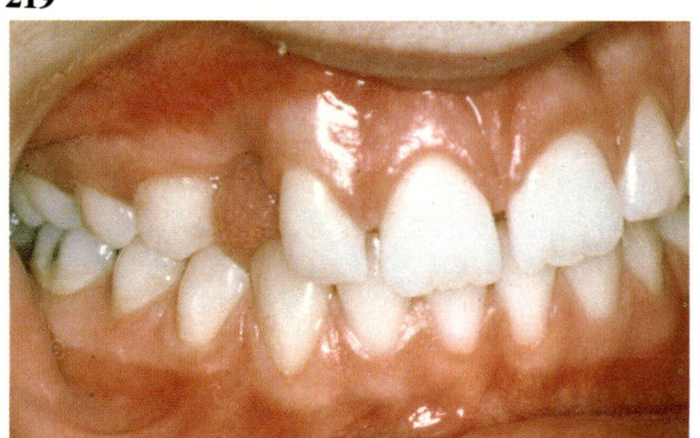

219 Intraoral view showing spacing of anterior teeth.

220

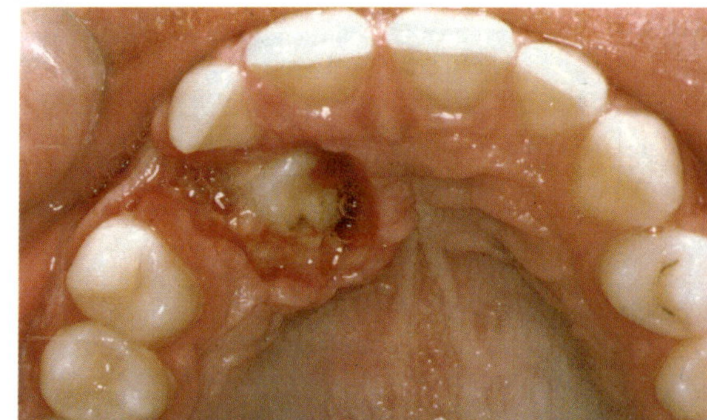

220 Occlusal view immediately after removal of the surgical pack, 10 days after surgical exposure of the canine.

221

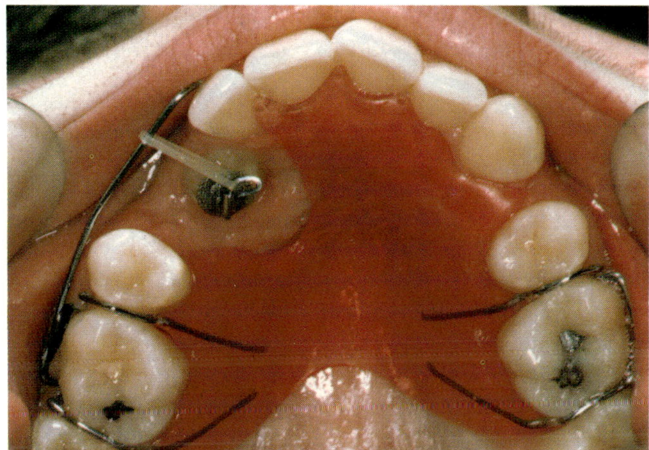

222

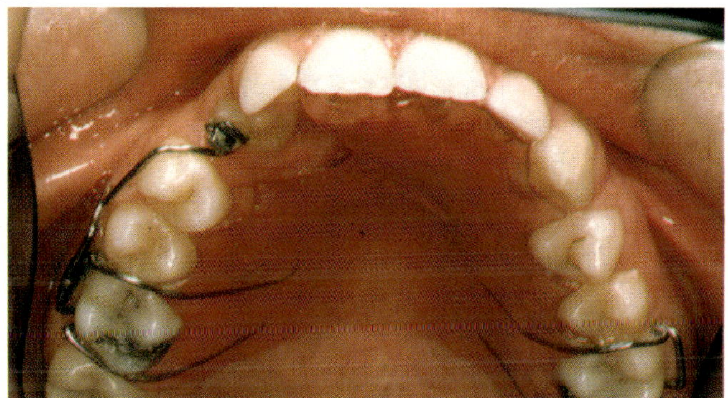

221 Occlusal view shows the use of a latex elastic from a bond on the upper right canine to a buccal wire on a removable appliance (different patient). A Begg bracket and brass pin have been used to make placement and removal of the elastic easier for the patient.

222 As the canine approaches the line of the arch, the elastic force becomes too small and the buccal wire can be adapted to engage the bracket directly.

223

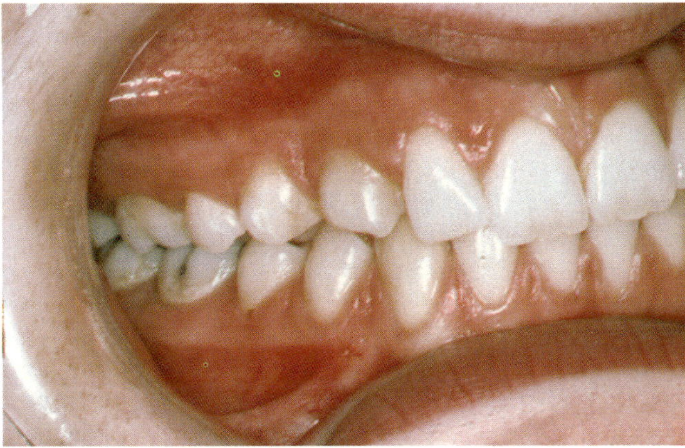

224

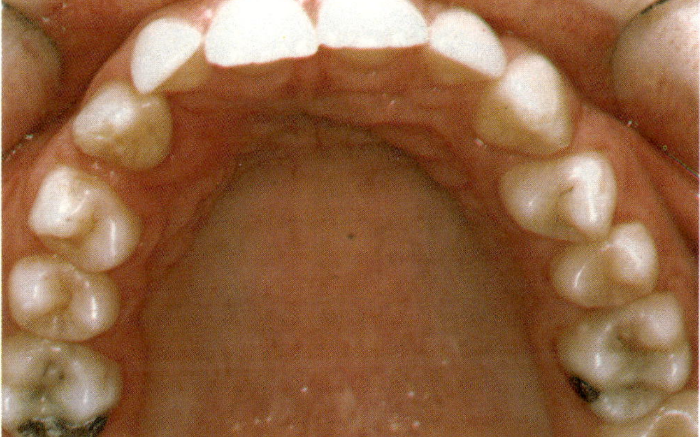

223 The canine is now in the line of the arch but not perfectly aligned.

224 Occlusal view shows the rotation of the canine. Further treatment was necessary to correct this.

225

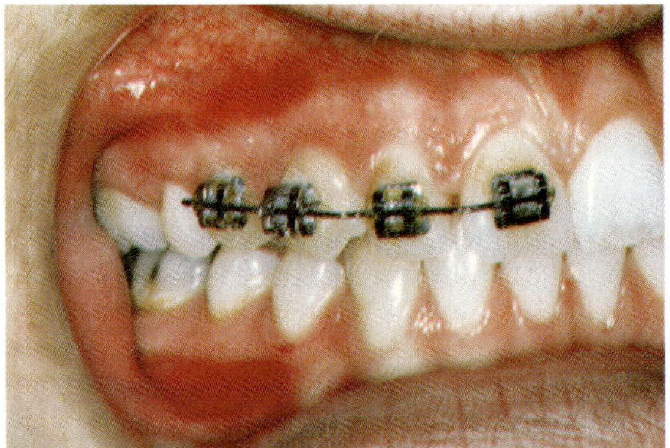

225 Simple fixed appliance in position labially. The original palatal bond has been removed.

226

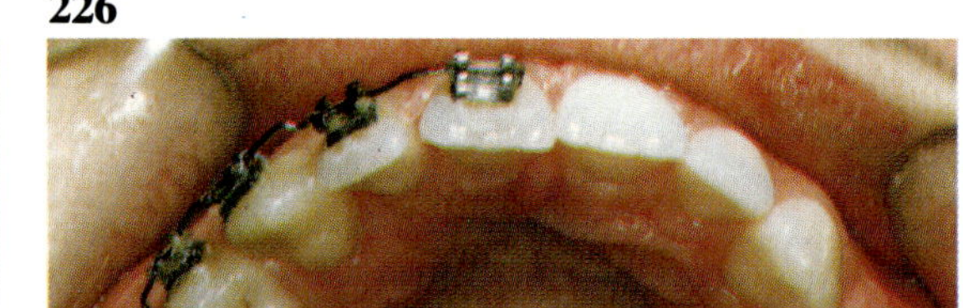

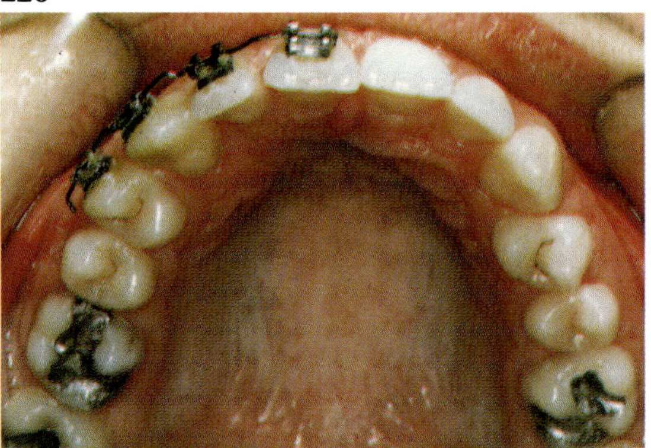

226 Occlusal view shows archwire bends.

227

227 Facial appearance with partially bonded appliance.

228

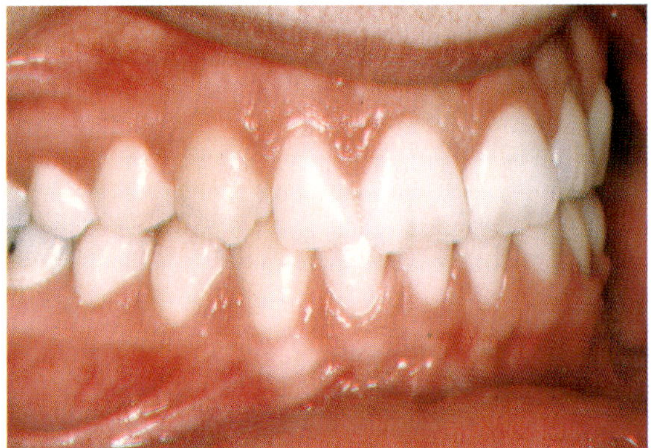

228 Occlusion after removal of the fixed appliance.

229

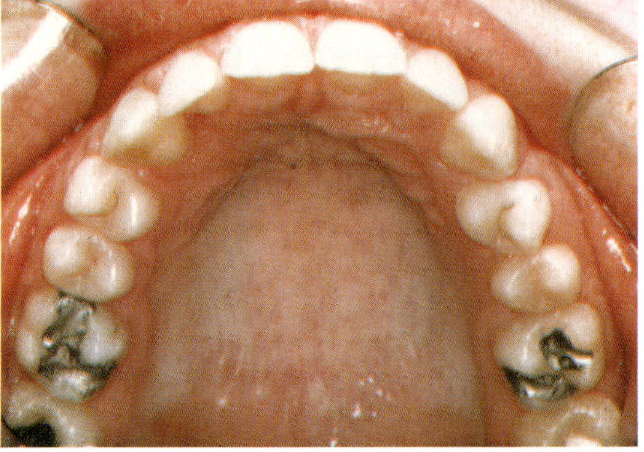

229 Occlusal view shows the corrected position of the upper right canine.

230

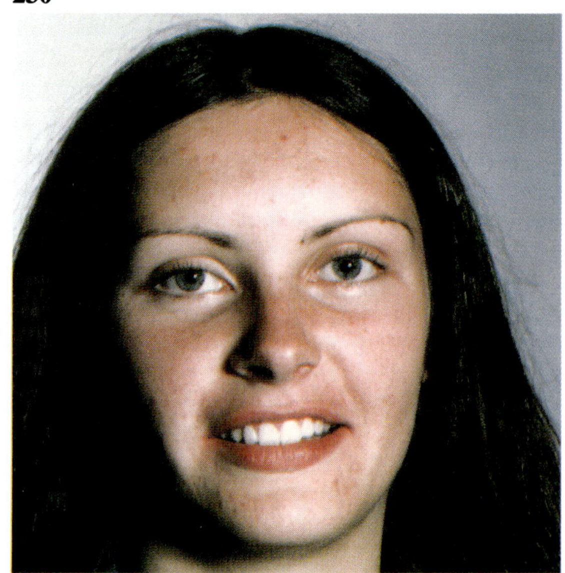

230 Facial view after removal of the appliance.

Removal of orthodontic brackets

Unlike fissure sealants and composite restorations, orthodontic brackets and their adhesive must be removed at the end of treatment. After removal of the arch wire, the brackets are removed easily but usually most of the composite material remains attached to the enamel. It has been remarked that the change from banding to bonding has transferred the most time-consuming procedure from the beginning to the end of treatment.

231

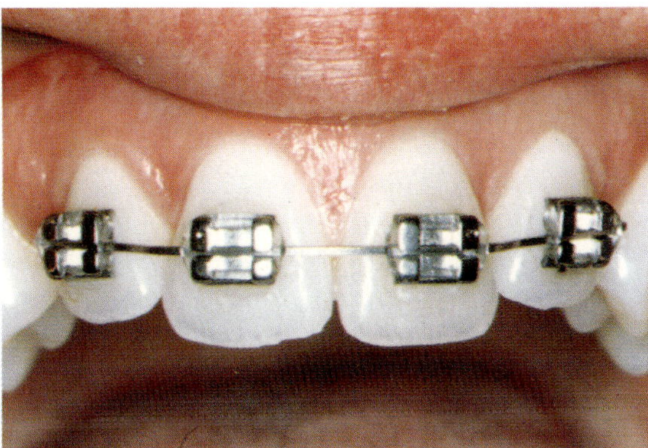

231 Appliance ready for removal. These brackets had been in position for five months. The arch wire is removed first.

232

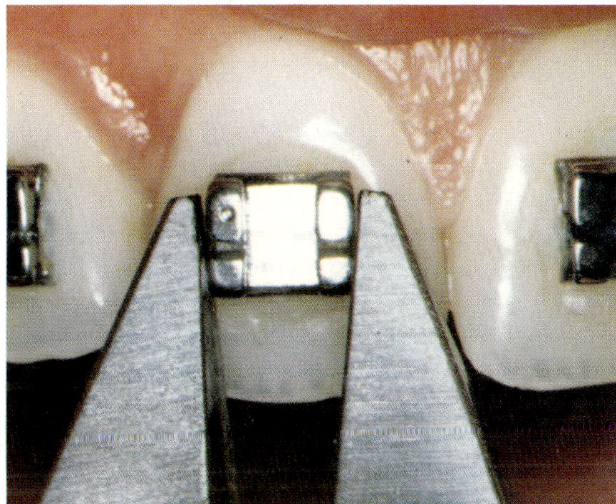

232 Perhaps the easiest way to remove this type of bracket is to squeeze it with a heavy pair of pliers until the back of the bracket distorts.

233

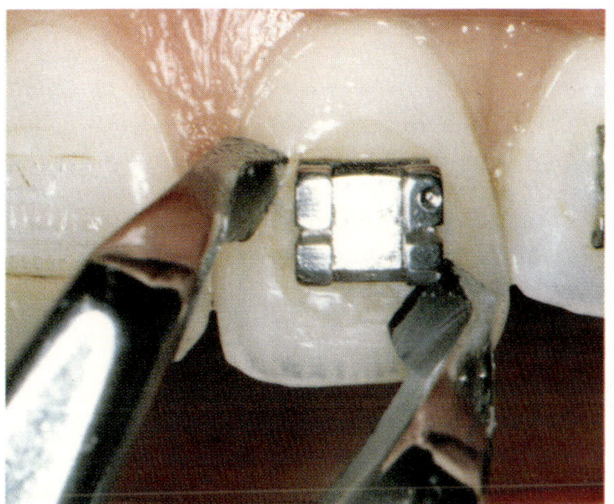

233 Another method is to use special bond removing pliers. Their cutting edges are applied to the back of the bracket base.

234

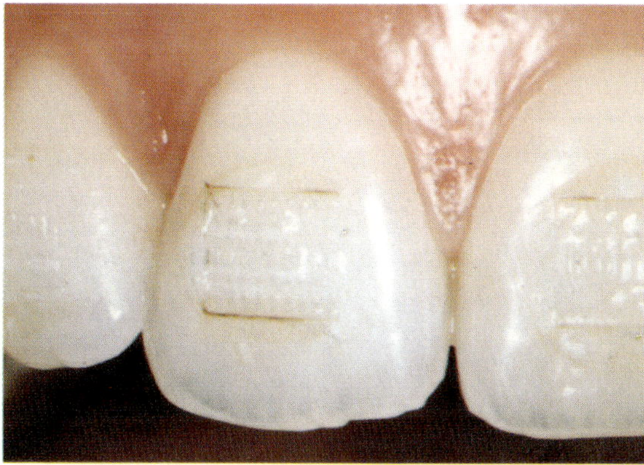

234 Most of the composite material has remained attached to the enamel surface demonstrating that the enamel/adhesive bond was stronger than the mechanical attachment of the adhesive to the bracket base.

235

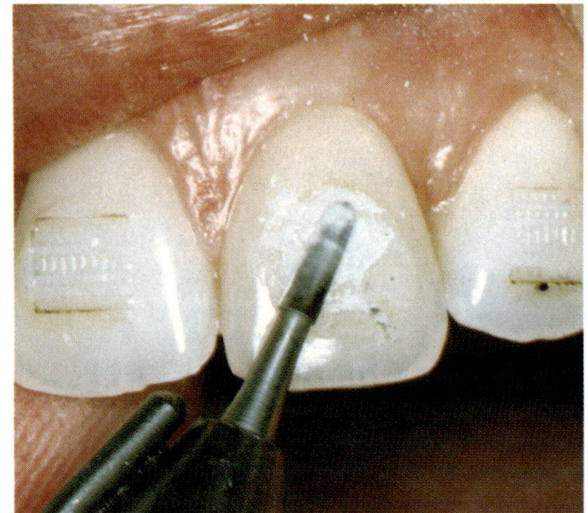

235 Removal of composite with a slowly revolving tungsten carbide bur. This is an efficient method, leaving a good enamel surface, but the bur soon becomes blunt.

236

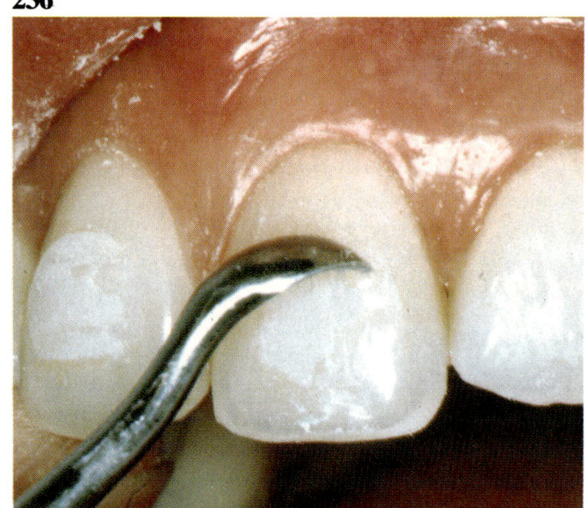

236 It is often possible to remove the last of the composite material with a scaler, but the enamel surface can be gouged even with a hand instrument if heavy pressure is used.

237

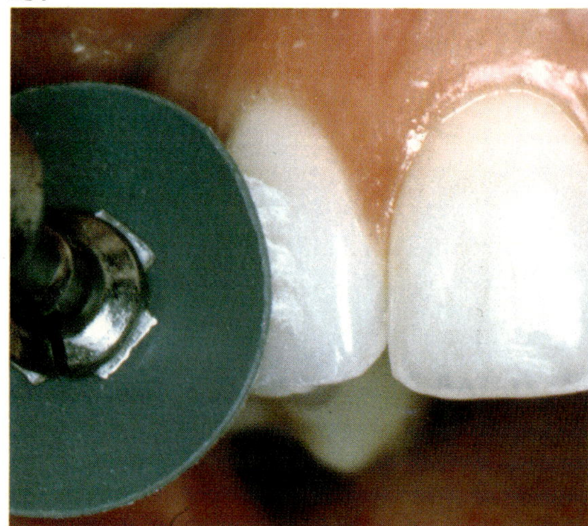

237 Flexible abrasive discs may be used but it is easy to scratch the enamel surface. Marks remain, even after the use of successively finer discs.

238

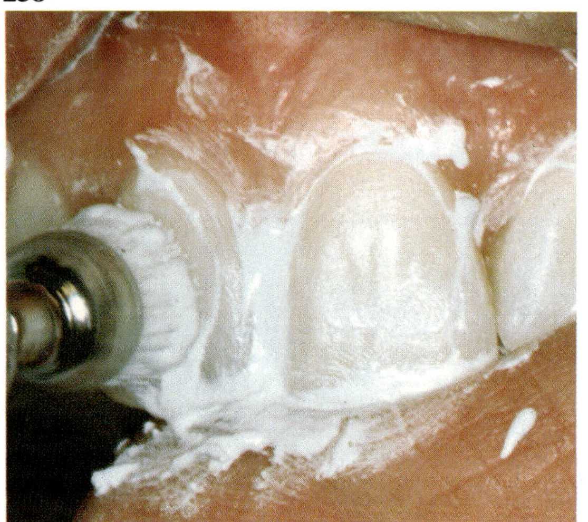

238 Final polishing of enamel surfaces.

239

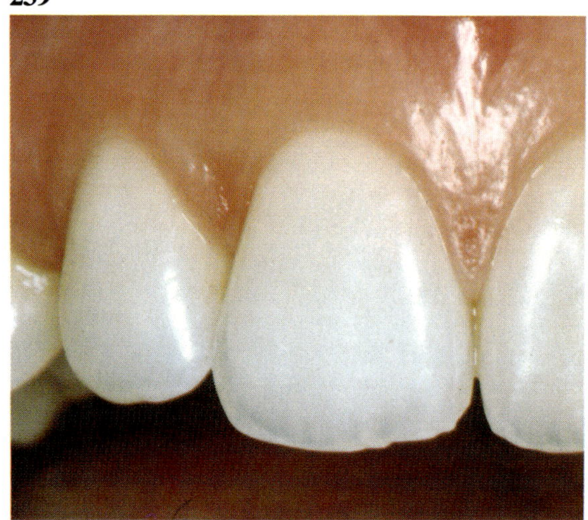

239 Resultant tooth surfaces.

Retention of orthodontic result

The more precisely teeth are aligned, the greater the need for them to be retained in their new positions. Rotations especially are notorious for their tendency to relapse and as much attention must be paid to the retention phase as to the active phase of treatment. Ideally some overcorrection of a rotation should have been carried out but this is not always easy to produce in practice.

The most positive retainer is the appliance which produced the tooth movement and it is a good idea to leave it in situ as a passive retainer for two or three months.

Traditionally, the fixed appliance was then removed and replaced by a removable retainer, worn full time for three months and then 12 hours a day, or nights only, to complete at least one year of retention. Severe rotations may justify even longer retention.

The development of direct bonding has enabled retention to be accomplished without a removable appliance, at least where only one or two teeth are to be retained. A wire may be bonded to the labial surfaces of adjacent teeth near the gingival margin or in many cases it is possible to bond onto the palatal surfaces, provided the occlusion permits.

240

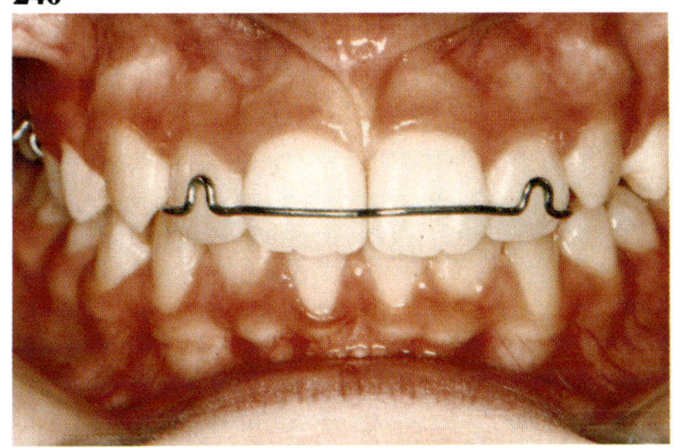

240 Traditional removable retainer, retaining upper left central incisor.

241

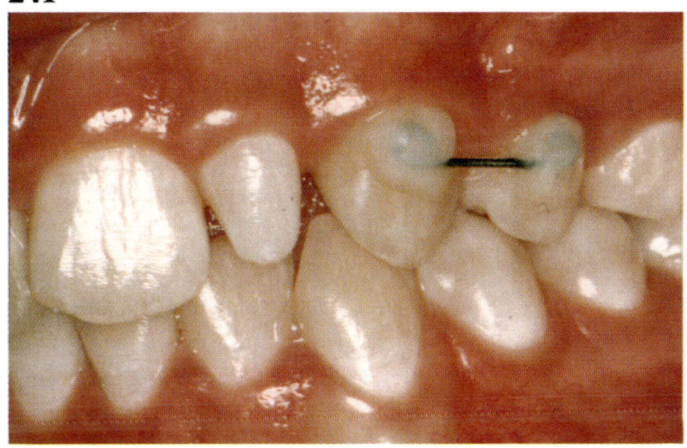

241 Wire bonded to the labial surfaces of $\lfloor 34$ after rotation of $\lfloor 3$ with a whip spring. The wire is visible but not very conspicuous.

242

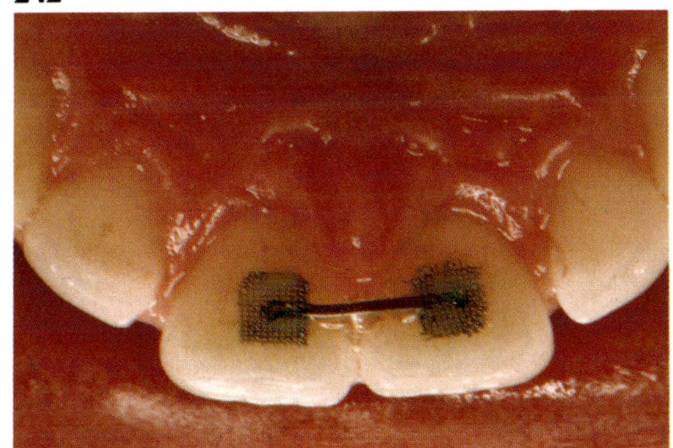

242 Wire and gauze pads used to retain $\underline{1|1}$ after rotation.

243

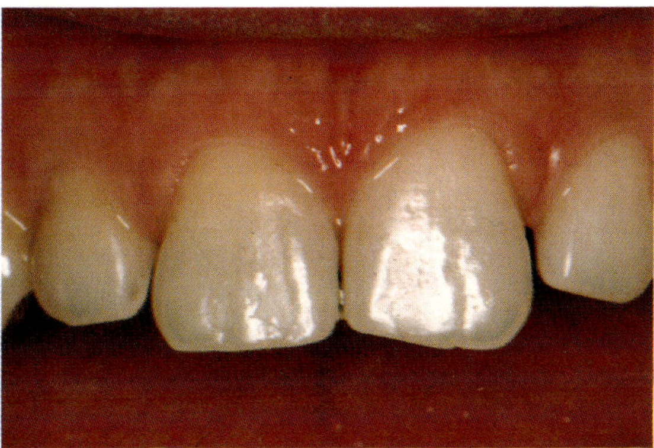

243 Labial view of the same patient.

Conclusion

In the preceding pages we have tried to trace some of the clinical developments in the acid etch technique over the last 10 to 15 years. There is no doubt that the ability to bond dental materials directly onto enamel has enlarged considerably the range of clinical procedures in paedodontics and orthodontics. Every clinical procedure is subject to development and the acid etch technique is no exception. We hope that this book will encourage dentists to widen their range of clinical skills and that they will adapt and improve our suggestions in the light of their own clinical experience and of developments reported in the current dental literature.

Throughout the chapters we have tended to follow the manufacturers' recommendations in suggesting etching for 60 seconds, washing for 10 to 30 seconds, and drying for up to 30 seconds. Some studies have suggested that much shorter etching times are equally effective in the application of fissure sealants. This possibility should be remembered because it would make fissure sealing even more acceptable to young and sometimes apprehensive patients.

Considerable attention has been given to the appearance of orthodontic appliances. Bonded metal brackets are much more acceptable aesthetically than orthodontic bands, but they are still conspicuous and this can be a problem to older patients especially. Plastic brackets are much less conspicuous when placed but plastic replicas of metal brackets fractured easily and were subject to deformation and creep when heavier forces were used. In addition, the original plastic brackets discoloured badly in the mouth. Better polycarbonate resins were developed, and stronger but more bulky designs were produced; even so, plastic brackets have not proved to be as popular as originally expected. Metal brackets have been made smaller and are used in most cases, with plastic brackets being reserved for upper anterior teeth in adult patients for whom limited tooth movements are to be carried out.

A recent development in the quest for the invisible orthodontic appliance is the 'lingual orthodontic appliance' in which brackets are bonded to the lingual or palatal surfaces of the teeth. The technique is not fully developed and has its difficulties; it too may prove to be best reserved for selected adult patients.

We have deliberately made no reference to specific papers or articles in the book to keep the text as simple as possible, in what is essentially a practical book aimed at the 'first-time user'. However, a selected bibliography is provided for further reading.

Bibliography

Books

The Acid Etch Technique – Proceedings of an International Symposium, Editors: Silverstone, L.M. & Dogon, I.L. North Central Pub. Co., St Paul, Minnesota, 1975.

Clinical Application of the Acid-Etch Technique Simonsen, R.J., Quintessence Publishing Co. Inc., Chicago, 1978.

Traumatic Injuries of the Teeth, Andreasen, J.O., (2nd edition) Munksgaard, Copenhagen, 1981.

Introduction to Fixed Appliances, Isaacson, K.G. & Williams, J.K. (3rd edition) Dental Practitioner Handbook No. 17, Wright, P.S.G., Bristol, 1984.

Articles

Buonocore, K.G. (1970): 'Adhesive sealing of pits and fissures for caries prevention, with use of ultraviolet light.' *J. Am. Dent. Ass.,* **80,** 324–8.

Cueto, E.I. & Buonocore, M.G. (1967): 'Sealing of pits and fissures with an adhesive resin: its use in caries prevention.' *J. Am. Dent. Ass.,* **75,** 121–8.

Faunce F.R. (1977): 'Tooth restoration with preformed laminate veneers.' *Dental Survey,* 30–32.

Horowitz, H.S. (1980): 'Pit and fissure sealants in private practice and public health programmes: an analysis of cost-effectiveness.' *Int. Dent. J.,* **30,** 117–26.

Horowitz, H.S. Heifetz, S.B., & Poulson, S. (1977): 'Retention and effectiveness of a single application of an adhesive sealant in preventing dental caries: final report after five years of a study in Kalispell, Montana.' *J. Am. Dent. Ass.,* **95,** 1133–9.

Livaditis, G.J. and Thompson, V.P. (1982): 'Etched Castings: An improved retentive mechanism for resin-bonded retainers.' *J. Prosthet. Dent.,* **47,** 52–58.

Raadal, M. (1978): 'Microleakage around preventive composite fillings in occlusal fissures.' *Scan J. Dent. Res,* **86,** 495–499.

Reynolds, I.R. (1975): 'A review of direct orthodontic bonding.' *Brit. J. Orthod.,* **2,** 171–178.

Roberts, G.J. (1983): 'Mastique Acrylic Laminate Veneers.' *Br. Dent. J.,* **155,** 85–88.

Rochette A.L. (1973): 'Attachment of a split to enamel of lower anterior teeth.' *J. Prosthet. Dent.,* **30,** 418–423.

Rock, W.P., Gordon, P.H. & Bradnock, G. (1978): 'The effect of operator variability and patient age on the retention of fissure sealant resin.' *Br. Dent. J.,* **145,** 232–4.

Simonsen, R.J. (1980): 'Preventive resin restorations: three year result.' *J. Am. Dent. Ass.,* **100,** 535–539.

Stephen, K.W., Kirkwood, M., Main, C. Gillespie, F.C. & Campbell, D. (1982): 'Retention of a filled fissure sealant using reduced etch time.' *Br. Dent. J.,* **153,** 232–233.

Zachrisson, B.U. (1977): 'A post-treatment evaluation of direct bonding in orthodontics.' *Am. J. Orthod.,* **71,** 173–189.

Zachrisson, B.U. & Arthun, J. (1979): 'Enamel surface appearance after various debonding techniques.' *Am. J. Orthod.,* **75,** 121–137

Index

All figures refer to page numbers